Student Success in
Medical School

T0127819

Student Success in Medical School

A Practical Guide to Learning Strategies

RAMAN MEHRZAD, MD, MHL, MBA

The Warren Alpert Medical School of Brown University,
Providence, RI

ELSEVIER

1600 John F. Kennedy Blvd.
Ste 1600
Philadelphia, PA 19103-2899

Content Strategist: Marybeth Thiel
Content Development Specialist: Marybeth Thiel
Publishing Services Manager: Deepthi Unni
Project Manager: Haritha Dharmarajan
Cover Designer: Patrick Ferguson

Printed in The United States of America

Last digit is the print number: 9 8 7 6 5 4 3 2 1

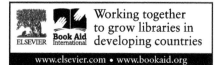

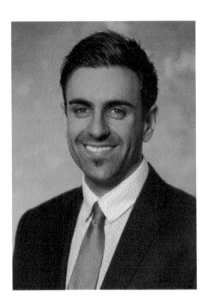

Raman Mehrzad, MD, MHL, MBA, is a physician, scientist, author, and educational expert. Born in Iran, Dr. Mehrzad moved to Sweden with his family at the age of 3, and then relocated to the United States after finishing medical school.

In 2015, he finished his residency training in internal medicine and began practising specialty medicine at Yale New Haven Hospital at the Yale School of Medicine, where he also became a medical director and clinical instructor for medical students and residents. He then re-specialized in plastic and reconstructive surgery and is currently a resident at The Warren Alpert Medical School of Brown University in Providence, Rhode Island. He has won the best medical student teaching award 2 years in a row at Brown University.

In conjunction with his work as a physician, Dr. Mehrzad also received an Executive Master of Healthcare Leadership from Brown University, as well as a Master of Business Administration from the Isenberg School of Management at the University of Massachusetts, graduating at the top of his class in both programs with a 4.0 GPA. He is a member of the honour society Phi Kappa Phi.

Dr. Mehrzad is the author of multiple books, runs three companies, and serves as a consultant for schools and businesses. His first book, *Straight A's: The Secret to Getting Top Grades in School*, became a bestseller in Sweden within its first week of sales and is currently available in five countries. Dr. Mehrzad has published several peer-reviewed articles in scientific journals and is currently pursuing clinical trials for a gene therapy drug that he and his research group have developed.

For any questions, comments, or other inquiries, please do not hesitate to contact Dr. Mehrzad by email (raman_m1@hotmail.com) or through his website or social media channels:

www.RamanMehrzad.com
LinkedIn: Raman Mehrzad
Instagram: @RamanMehrzad
TikTok: RamanMehrzad
Facebook: Raman Mehrzad

Medicine is a fascinating, challenging, and fulfilling field in which to pursue a career. It is also a diverse and rapidly evolving field that will stay relevant for as long as humans exist. As a physician, you will not only be rewarded personally and professionally, you will also be given the opportunity to improve the well-being of individuals, communities, and society as a whole. As a new medical school graduate, you will find that the job market is stable, the income potential is high, and the career satisfaction also tends to be high. For these reasons, admission to medical school is highly competitive and requires excellent grades, high MCAT scores, and significant individual merits on your curriculum vitae. Moreover, successfully graduating from medical school and entering more competitive specialties is far from easy.

What makes for a successful medical student? Most students go in "blindly" without knowing how to prepare in advance or what to expect. Preparation in life is key and one of the most important factors to achieving greatness in anything. If you *know* what to do and *when* to do it in advance, it will be much easier to excel in your performance, rather than learning through trial and error as you go along. Thus, you need a strategy and a systematic approach to each and every course and clinical rotation.

The routines of daily life are mostly based on a system, even if that system is unconscious at times. When you get up in the morning, you have a system in how to prepare yourself for school or work. For instance, you might turn off the alarm clock (step 1), jump into the shower (step 2), get dressed (step 3), eat your breakfast (step 4), gather your personal belongings (step 5), walk out the door to head to your destination (step 6), and so on. You have a methodical approach to most things in life. This is also the case in business where you have stepwise processes (process flow). This methodical approach has been shown to not only add structure but also efficiency to processes, since you know what to do and when to do it.

In school, however, methodical and efficient processes are not always a given. Students get thrown into a class without actually knowing what, when, and how to do things in a systematic routine. Some students will figure it out quickly, while others never do. This ability to "figure it out" could make the difference between success and failure.

This book is the first comprehensive, evidence-based guide on how to excel in medical school. With this book, you will get all the information you need on how to motivate yourself, strategize, build an accurate plan, set goals, do well on lectures, and manage your time. Furthermore, you will learn about some of the best learning and study techniques for this field in particular; these techniques will not just optimize your learning, but also show you exactly what to do in each and every course. Put simply, this is the guide you need in order to perform well and come out on top in medical school—to know what, when, and how to do things from day one.

Remember that many students who do well in medical school are not geniuses—they just figured out the system. With this book, you will learn exactly that: the system on how to succeed and hopefully be much better prepared than others.

CONTENTS

Student Success in
Medical School

Key Factors to Success in School

Introduction to Success in Medical School

Your Future, Your Choices

Buckle up, dear student, because this is an aggressively honest chapter. You won't find any sugar-coated sentiments here. This is where I tell you how you can optimize your success in medical school and achieve your dreams. I am going to share with you the reality of how success works in any venture. If you really want to succeed in medical school and match into your specialty of choice, you must be prepared to work hard and persevere.

You Don't Have to Be a Genius to Succeed

You don't have to be the smartest person in the world to reach the top. I'm no slouch, but I'm no Einstein either. Nevertheless, I've achieved great things in my life starting at a young age. And if I could do it, so can you.

I got into medical school at 19, finished a semester before anyone else in my class, wrote my first book when I was 21, started my first company when I was 22, came to America and matched into plastic surgery, and have published extensively. I have two master's degrees in addition to my MD, all of which I completed with a 4.0 grade point average. (To mention a few accomplishments.) How did I do all this? By having a strong will, working hard, and cultivating key qualities (more on that below). That is one major difference between me and most people: my strong will. Everyone who knows me knows that I make things happen. I am a man of action. If I want something, I go for it, and I do whatever it takes to get there. Whenever I find myself in a challenging situation, my thought process goes like this: "You can be smarter and more talented than me, but you will never defeat me—because you do not have my hunger, my drive, and my ability to set goals and reach them." You need to develop that same mindset.

There is no single quality that has determined my success. Success demands vision, drive, hard work, perseverance, patience, confidence, determination, curiosity, an open mind, diligence, discipline, strategic thinking, ambition, integrity, passion, self-reliance, and optimism. It means sleepless nights, a lot of sweat, and many tears. Yes, the list of qualities you need is long, and the road to success is longer still. But I'm here to tell you that I've been there *and* that I promise you that this massive effort will be worth it. I also promise you that if you work hard, it won't just help you in medical school but also in life.

If you want to succeed, then you must first *want* to succeed. Most other things in your life should not matter. Who you are, how smart you are, what your background is—none of it matters. You should focus only on thinking about your goals and striving to reach them. And trust me: It's almost impossible to defeat someone who has their eyes on their goals and never gives up!

Do you think I was the smartest of all the thousands that applied for a plastic surgery residency, the most competitive specialty in medicine? No way! I competed with the best medical students and physicians from the best schools in the United States and around the world. We are talking about people with high IQs and intelligence, the most ambitious medical students and physicians with the best qualifications behind them.

Studying for the medical licensing exams and applying for residency meant that I had to endure one demanding exam after another, one administrative process after another, and one interview after another. I knew I would be competing with the best in the field. And yes, I cried. Yes, I was stressed. Yes, I was sleep deprived. I probably didn't eat as much as I should have. It was extremely tough, rough, and difficult. But I never gave up and I didn't let anyone, or anything, scare me. The truth is that I don't really care if someone has a thousand more qualifications than me—they will never have my hunger.

Many people tried to discourage me from chasing my dreams, but I never let them get to me. I didn't let the thought of how difficult or competitive the process was scare me. And you should not let these things scare you either. You should never let people discourage you. If you haven't already learned this about people, allow me to enlighten you now: People will hate you for no reason. They will let you down, they will discourage you, they may even betray you. They will make you feel angry, sad, afraid—you name it! But you need to be strong minded, tough, and never let them get to you. Call it motivation, inspiration, or a driving force. You have one life and you deserve to get the best out of it. Don't let anyone stop you.

Your Future is Determined by You

Your future is determined by you alone. It's not determined by anyone or anything else: not your circumstances, not your background, not who your parents were. There is one key factor within your control that will determine your future: how bad you want it. If you want something bad enough, you will always find a way. Some things will come easy in life, while other things will not. And if you want those things, you have to work for them. Big goals, such as getting into medical school and matching into a competitive residency, don't come easy. You really have to want it. It is not enough to want it just a little bit. You have to want to succeed so much that everything else comes second.

With this foundation laid, I will now tell you a story about success.

There was a young man who wanted to make a lot of money, so he went to visit a guru. He told the guru, "I want to be on the same level that you're on." And so the guru replied, "If you want to be on the same level that I'm on, meet me here tomorrow at the beach at 4 am." The man thought, *The beach? I said I want to make money, I don't want to swim.* But the young man did as he was told and arrived at the beach at 4 am, ready to do whatever it took. The old guru grabbed his head. "How bad do you want to be successful?" "Real bad," replied the man. So the guru said, "Walk out into the water." So the man walked out into the water until it was waist deep. He thought to himself, *This man's crazy. I want to make money, and he's got me out here swimming! I didn't ask to be a lifeguard. I want to make money.* The guru said, "Come out a little farther." So the man did. The water was now up to his shoulders. He thought to himself, *This old guru is crazy. He's making money, but he's crazy.* The guru said, "Come out a little farther." The man again came out a little farther. The water was now up to his mouth. The young man said, "I'm getting out. You are out of your mind." But the guru shouted, "I thought you wanted to be successful?!" He said, "I do! But this is ridiculous!" The guru said, "Walk a little farther." The guru then approached the man and pushed his head underwater. The guru held the man down under the water. The man was scratching, clawing, and fighting to get up. The guru continued to hold him down underwater. Then, just before the young man was about to pass out, the guru grabbed him under the arms and lifted him up. The man began gasping for air. The guru looked the young man right in the eyes and said, "Now tell me something. When you were underwater, what was the only thing you wanted to do, more than anything?" The young man shouted, "I wanted to breathe!" The guru said, "Exactly. When you want to succeed as bad as you want to breathe, then you'll be successful."

Have you ever had trouble breathing? Or had a panic or anxiety attack? You may have aspirated on a piece of food or had an asthma attack. If you have ever temporarily lacked the ability to breathe normally, then you know that the only thing you wanted in those situations was to breathe. When you cannot breathe, you don't care about what happened yesterday, what will happen tomorrow, who did you wrong, who did you right, what clothes to wear next week, or anything else. All you want to do is live. So you will do anything in your power to breathe. All your focus and energy goes to finding a way to help you breathe.

You have to apply that same mentality to achieving success. When you get to a point in your life where the only thing you want is to be successful, and when you want that success as badly as taking a single breath, then that day you are guaranteed to be successful.

You Have to Prioritize

I sometimes hear students say that they want higher grades, that they want to get into a specific competitive residency program, or that they want to make a lot of money in the future. However, the problem is often that they do not want it badly enough. They do not want it as badly as partying, having friends, watching movies, or playing videogames. But if you really want to be successful, you have to sacrifice. You have to put aside friends, partying, videogames, TV, and social media. Sometimes you may even have to sacrifice sleep or meals!

Does that sound tough? It is! Did you think being successful was easy? Did you think getting into the top residency programs was a piece of cake? Did you think making a lot of money, staying healthy, and getting a good job were things that you could do without sacrificing things in life? If so, then you're mistaken. If it were that easy, everybody would do it.

Some may find the things I say harsh or even exaggerated. But most people who succeed in life will agree with me and tell you that these things are true. Successful people know that a strong will and hard work are required if you want to achieve big things. Hardly anyone gets things handed to them. You get what you work for. As professional basketball player Damian Lillard said, "If you want to look good in front of thousands, you have to outdo thousands in front of nobody."

Remember that sacrifices will be required at times. But these sacrifices are only temporary. Pain is only temporary. If you want to succeed, you sometimes have to endure tough times and be okay with that. The reward for your work will come later. You will have so many wonderful moments once you have achieved your goal—especially if you get to do what you dream of doing *every single day.*

There Are No Shortcuts to Success

I laugh at those who think you can succeed, earn good grades, and get positive evaluations without working hard. It's not just a lie, it's propaganda. You can't be successful by leaning back and doing things at the last moment. There are no excuses for laziness. Success begins in your mind with your mentality, your way of thinking. This is where you lay the groundwork to grow as a human, build on your merits, and ultimately fulfill your dreams. But it takes time, planning, dedication, intelligence, ambition, the right thinking, the right attitude, and a lot of hard work to achieve it. And the faster you adopt this way of thinking, the better. It is only then that you really will spend the time required and do whatever it takes to get wherever you want without it being that difficult for you. It will not be easy, but I can promise you two things. One, it is *not* impossible to achieve your goals and dreams. And two, I promise you that it will be worth it! Ambition nearly always beats talent.

You Can Overcome Laziness and Build a Winning Mentality

Are you a lazy person? Do you wonder if you can ever adopt a winning mentality? Do you scratch your head and wonder if you can work as hard as I'm saying you have to? Well, I can tell you that you definitely can. You can build a winning mentality, overcome your laziness, and develop a stronger will and be more ambitious by doing three things: (1) get the knowledge, (2) want it, and (3) practice it. Just like you learned how to crawl, walk, and run by practicing when you were a baby, you can develop all these other traits as well. You can be better at everything by gaining the necessary knowledge, wanting it, and practicing it.

As a physician, I often have to convince patients with diabetes, high blood pressure, and cardiovascular disease that they need to change their lifestyles so they can live longer. In the same way, I am now asking you to change your mentality so that you have a better future. A slacking attitude in school or life is not compatible with success. If a diabetic patient can understand their situation, then you should be able to understand yours, right?

Imagine you are at a crossroads. One road is gritty with many uphill slopes but leads to a good goal. The other is straight and sunny but leads to a bad goal. Which road would you take? I am sure you wouldn't choose the one that leads to a bad goal just because it is sunnier and easier to walk that road, right? Of course, you would take the more difficult route that leads you where you want to go. Unfortunately, if you choose an easier life now, you will likely end up having a harder time later on. But if you choose to go through some hardship now, you will most likely have a much easier and better time down the road.

Laziness is a feeling that can sometimes be hard to beat, but it can be overcome with a little bit of willpower. As soon as something feels hard to you, you should tell yourself, "This is just a feeling, and I should not let a feeling take over my future!" Today, there may be many things that you do not feel like doing. But once you reach your goals, the tables will turn so that you can do exactly what you want most of the time.

Are you going to let a fleeting feeling determine your life, knowingly throwing away opportunities for a better future? Think about it and consciously change yourself now. If you change your mindset, everything will change. But if you don't change, then nothing changes.

In the End, We Only Regret the Chances We Did Not Take

Jim Rohn once said, "We must all suffer one of two things: the pain of discipline or the pain of regret and disappointment." Throughout my career, I've heard many physicians and medical students say, "Oh I wish I had studied harder in school and gotten better evaluations and scores." You probably also know people that wish they had worked harder. It could be your parents, a relative, or someone else living with the knowledge that they could have a completely different life if they had just worked harder.

Remember that we do not regret the things that we do but rather the things that we didn't do. You do not want to end up in a situation where you wish you had worked harder but didn't. So take this information into your heart and understand that working hard now will keep you from waking up when you're 50, filled with regret and wishing you had done things differently.

By contrast, if you ask people who did work really hard in school and ended up succeeding, they will say that it was the best choice they ever made. They will say it was worth all the sleepless nights and sweat and tears, that the road to get there was hard, but it was worth the struggle. And I promise that you will say the same thing in 10 years if you follow my advice.

Take a Deep Breath and Be Calm

What I've said might be overwhelming and come across as too intense. (I did warn you that this is an aggressive chapter.) But also remember that I am here to give you the truth in order to help you. I am here to give you the roadmap to success. I am not here to tell you things that won't work. You have invested in this book, and my goal is to give you information that pays for itself a thousand times over. It is therefore my intention to share with you only those things that work. Things that many successful people know and do every day. I will not sit here and tell you that you can chill out and still become a plastic surgeon in 4 years.

Take it one day at a time. Rome was not built in a day, and you are not becoming chief of surgery tomorrow! All you should think about right now is building a winning mentality and practicing it every day. As long as you have the will and work hard, I promise that the rest will come to you eventually. You don't need to know exactly how to get to your goals right now. You will see that the road will clear out the more you walk it. As Martin Luther King said, "You don't have to see the whole staircase, just take the first step." You don't need to know exactly how to get to your goal—few people do. It is just enough to really want to get there. The road will then become clear for you. Trust me!

Think Positive and Start From Day One

As you should realize by now, it takes a lot to succeed in medical school (and in life). Sometimes it will get really tough. But always keep your head high and never give up. You know what your reward is later. You know what benefits a high score on the USMLEs and good evaluations are for your residency applications. And you know what opportunities you will have access to as a result. Therefore, get ready to fight until you reach your goal, and don't stop a second before that. These are going to be your best years, the years that you will build the amazing things that you will enjoy for the rest of your life.

Make sure you start today. Do not wait until tomorrow or next month. Important things tend to slip through the cracks if we don't grab hold of them right away. Therefore, begin to prepare yourself mentally to fight for success starting from day one. Clear your thoughts of everything negative and think positive. This chapter is meant to inspire you and help you muster the energy and courage you need. Now, sit back and think about how nice it will feel to do something you never thought possible. This moment is the start of something big.

CHAPTER 2

The Art of Studying in the Medical Field

I didn't come this far to come only this far.
— Tom Brady

Introduction

You made it to medical school—congratulations! You have accomplished something that many dream of doing but few actually do. Medicine is an amazing field. You get to learn how the body works, how diseases occur, how to manage and treat various conditions, and how to help people with the most important aspect of life: health and well-being. But studying in medical school is different from studying in other fields. There is a massive amount of information to learn in a short time. You will engage in a combination of theoretical and practical learning. You will have clinical rotations, be tested through written and practical exams, and be forced to use your theoretical and social knowledge and skills in order to succeed.

As I mentioned at the outset, you obviously didn't come this far to only get this far. Getting into medical school is difficult, but this is just the start of your career. The better you do in medical school, the better your chances of having a successful career. In this chapter, I will explain the most important differences between medical school and other programs and educate you about the challenges and opportunities so that you are well informed, know how to build a positive mentality, and can better position yourself for success.

Differences Between Medicine and Other Fields

The first and most obvious difference is that you are learning human biology in its entirety, from cells and molecules all the way up to organ systems and the human body as a whole. There is a lot of information that will be thrown at you. And it's not just the volume of learning that can be overwhelming; it's also the depth and complexity of it.

Becoming a physician requires a good understanding of anatomy, histology, cell biology, chemistry, physiology, and many other subjects. It's not like other fields where you can learn a formula, calculate a problem, and then move on to the next question. For instance, figuring out differential diagnoses can be tricky and does not always follow the "textbook" approach. The only way to be a good diagnostician is to have a detailed understanding of how the body works. To do so, you'll have to spend a lot of time reading and rereading information until it both sticks in your brain and you have a fundamental understanding of it[1-3].

First, you'll start with the basics: nomenclature. You need to know the proper name for every part of the body, where each part is located, and how the parts interact with each other. The names of body parts are one thing. The names of different structures and the different parts of each structure, as well as how they relate to each other, is another. You are learning a new language. In medicine, communication is universal and needs to be the same no matter where we are in the world. By learning anatomy, histology, and other core courses, you will develop this foundation of knowledge[1,2].

Second, you need to know how different cells, organs, and tissues work and what they do. Fortunately (or unfortunately), cells, organs and tissues do not do just one thing. They often have multiple functions and interact with each other in the process. Therefore, you will learn how cells divide and how DNA is copied during cell division. You will learn how cells die and why they do. You will learn what happens if cells don't die (as they should) and what this problem could lead to. Moving up to the next level of complexity, you will learn how cells and tissues should look (morphology and histology) and also how they'll look if they are subjected to an injury or an internal or external stressor. Next, you will learn the functionality of different organs. Why do we have a heart? What does the spleen do? Why can't we live without a liver? How can we live with just one kidney? All these questions have amazing and interesting answers that you will learn in depth[1-3].

Once you learn the basics of how the human body works and what different structures look like and are called, you'll then continue by learning what could happen when something goes wrong in the body and why, otherwise known as pathology. Pathology is the science of the causes and effects of different diseases. You will learn the difference between a stroke and a myocardial infarction (often incorrectly referred to as a heart attack). You will understand why a bacterial infection may need to be treated with antibiotics and why viruses are not. Only once you've arrived at this step will you actually start learning about what many physicians deal with on a daily basis: identifying and understanding disease processes and then trying to manage or treat them. But as you can see, if you don't first gain fundamental knowledge about human biology, then learning pathology will be useless because you will not be able to completely understand it. You won't be able to comprehend why certain symptoms emerge during a disease state. Therefore, a complete understanding of cells, organs, tissues, and the human body as a whole is essential before you can start to diagnose common disorders[1,2].

Many other fields or programs do not require this depth of understanding to able to do the work later. Many other fields also do not have the same stepwise learning, where you need to learn step one before you can move on to (and understand) step two. In business school, you can learn about marketing first and then finance or vice versa. You can learn about business law first and then strategy or vice versa. The order doesn't make a difference. Moreover, even if you don't know all aspects of marketing, you will still be able to move on in your business career with a basic understanding (and fill in the gaps later)[4,5].

Therefore, my first and most essential piece of advice to you is to truly invest your time in learning the basics extremely well. And when I say extremely well, I mean to learn it so well that the knowledge becomes second nature to you. Many students question some of the courses and knowledge and ask why they need to know the minutiae of biochemical reactions when they are going to treat infections and wounds. The answer is simple: nearly all diseases have a physiological, biochemical, and/or cellular component. So if you do not know the actual mechanisms behind a disease, it will be tough to understand how disease states really work and to also remember how to manage different disorders. This initial investment will pay off greatly during your later years of medical school and in your career as a physician.

By contrast, if you don't learn the basics extremely well, you will have many issues later on. Trust me on this. I have seen too many physicians with suboptimal knowledge who are now struggling in their careers. You do not want to end up like that, as it may lead to severe negative consequences for you and your patients. If you learn just the bare minimum, those issues will translate to worse performance and worse grades in medical school.

Here is what I suggest to avoid this problem and to maximize your learning: If you don't understand something, read it again. And then again. Ask for help! Have a friend or your teacher explain it to you. If you don't remember something, repeat your learning through drills until you do. It's about working hard and putting in all the effort early on, during the first few years, to develop a fundamental knowledge about the human body and its inner workings. By learning things in depth, you will never go wrong[6].

Another challenging aspect of learning in medical school is balancing the learning process with trying to absorb the most important things. You have to understand that there is *so* much information in this field that you can spend your whole life studying and still never learn all there is to know. So when I say learn things well, I don't mean to learn 100% of all the details in every single course, because that would be impossible. There are things that are more and less important; you will figure out what information is most important, and your professor and course will guide you as to what those things are. It's about learning the essential things you need to get from one step to the next. Within the cell, for instance, you need to learn about DNA replication, different organelles and their functions, cell division, apoptosis, and so forth. But you may not need to spend weeks learning the role of cardiolipin concentration and acyl chain composition in the molecular organization and function of the mitochondrial inner membrane. The latter is just an example of how deep you can go into each aspect of the cell's structure and function; those details should be left to scientists who are pushing the field forward through specialized research[6].

Multiple Exams

In medical school, you will have many exams. Especially during the first couple of years. You may have two or three exams or quizzes *per week*[6]. Yes, testing could be that frequent. This is not a bad thing, however, since it pushes you to read and learn things at a faster pace. On the other hand, if you never had exams, you wouldn't feel the pressure of learning things quickly. However, this also means that you will feel the pressure and stress of relatively fast learning and be forced to perform well from the start. This fast pace of learning is one of the hardest things to adjust to at the beginning. Once orientation is over, you're "in business"—the business of sitting and reading for many hours every single day. First year will be all about memorizing the names of drugs, branches of blood vessels, nerves, bones, muscles, and so on. There will be lectures from morning until afternoon, and then solo studying the rest of the evening. That means long nights, managing your stress, and a constant battle of keeping yourself awake when you're tired.

Here are a few key points that you should remember from the start:

- Study from day one. Don't let a single day go by without doing the readings and reviewing your notes. Make sure you follow a study schedule and your plan without falling behind.
- Take notes on the lectures. Make sure you take good notes, since the things your professor brings up are typically the core of what you need to learn. You will need to learn other things as well, but this is the best approach to taking solid notes and also ensuring you have an easier time passing your weekly quizzes and exams.
- Have a system and strategy to learn. (This book will teach you how to do that.)

- On occasion, take a break from solo studying to study with a friend. Two brains can be better than one, so it's a good idea to sit with someone who you know learns things easily and can help you if there's something you don't understand. The key is to learn a lot in a short time.
- Battle the fatigue. You will be tired. You will fall asleep many times. You will feel like you just want to go to bed, but you have to stay awake. This is it. Remember: *You didn't come this far to only get this far.* The best way is to stick with the basics: work out a few times per week, eat healthy food, and get 6 to 7 hours of sleep. If you can't get that many hours, take power naps during the day. You could also drink coffee or tea (with small amounts of caffeine) to help you stay awake.

Multitasking

Medical school is all about multitasking. There are few programs out there that combine clinical work with theoretical studies the way medicine school does. You will begin clinical rotations after a short time. You'll have to balance rotations with lectures, studying, and classes. In addition, you need to study on your own. There are many things to fit into a day. You will learn how to make an accurate plan later in this book. Use that to structure your day, build a strategy, and execute it.

Learning Many Things Quickly

This may be one of the hardest things to deal with. We all get overwhelmed when there are thousands of things we need to learn and do it in a short time. You will feel that it's not doable. You will feel that you will never learn what you need to learn. You will feel that it's "impossible." All these feelings are normal and something that most medical students feel. Remember to take one day at a time. It's all about repetition, and soon you will get there just like everyone else before you. Just focus on learning the things you need to learn for the week and don't get too anxious about what's coming in the future. As long as you have a plan, stick to it, and work hard, you will most likely do fine.

Having said that, you need to boost your memorization skills, and this book will show you how you can memorize things in the most efficient way. You need to have the correct study techniques so that you learn things the right way from the start. This book will teach you how. Be aware that at times you will think to yourself, "This is impossible"; while it's normal to think that way, it certainly *is* possible!

Less Personal Life

Balancing medical school and a personal life is tough. Since time is of the essence and everyone has the same 24 hours each day, there will indeed be days when you cannot devote much time, if any, to a personal life. I assure you that once you have a system in place and get used to it, it will get better. However, in the beginning, you need to prepare yourself for the fact that there will be less time for friends, family, romantic relationships, exercise, and other personal activities. That is just the way it is. In life, we have to prioritize. When there isn't enough time, the most important things—the ones we assign the highest value to—often need to come first.

When you accept that you will have a challenging first year, you will feel less anxious and upset when you realize that you no longer have time for a personal life. In business, we call this opportunity cost[7], which is defined as the loss of potential gain from other alternatives when one option is chosen. An example of opportunity cost is when you spend 2 hours and $50 going out for dinner with a friend and now cannot spend that 2 hours at home studying nor that $50 on something else[7]. When we invest in something "difficult," such as studying for a biochemistry exam, and give up other "fun" stuff such as personal relationships, exercise, and entertainment, our investment in the thing we chose to do is the cost of not doing the fun stuff. This is just a part of this process. And there is not much you can do about it unless you are willing to compromise your learning and outcomes in medical school—which you should not. However, these sacrifices are just for a limited time. It's perfectly fine to temporarily give up certain things in life to invest in other things.

Having said that, you still need to cover basic self-care so that you can function well long term. We can all give up sleep, healthy eating habits, and exercise for a little while, but doing so long term will negatively affect your performance and health. Therefore, make sure that you sleep at least 6 hours per night. Try to exercise at least a couple of times per week. And do your best to eat nutritious food and avoid fast food and other empty calories. These habits are essential to your well-being and health and will impact your performance. Therefore, these basic acts of self-care should be prioritized. Sure, some days you will only be able to sleep 4 to 5 hours, and there will be weeks when you do not have time to go to the gym. However, these should be exceptions to the rule.

Delayed Gratification

Studying medicine and accomplishing the long-term dream of becoming a doctor takes time. In general, you have to do 4 years of pre-med, 4 years of medical school, and then at least 3 years of residency training[3-6] (the shortest residency training programs are 3 years). It's a long road ahead, and the road is bumpy. That is just the way it is. You are not signing up to learn how to assemble packages. You are learning how to save lives, so understand that your education at this stage requires a whole different dimension of learning, understanding, and doing, which means a long-term investment of your time and energy.

In medical school, you will not experience the immediate gratification that you would get with other programs that are shorter or in which there are more practical milestones to reach within the program's time frame[8]. This is just a fact you need to accept. Again, you are in a different program and field with many great benefits to come. However, to enjoy these benefits, you also have to accept the fact of delayed gratification. Patience is key, so keep it in mind at all times.

You will not be a practicing doctor after your first or second year of medical school. You may not even be an independent doctor after you graduate from medical school. In fact, many are not comfortable until after the first couple of years following graduate residency training, when they become attending physicians. Consequently, don't seek immediate gratification[8]. You're in this for the long haul with long-term benefits to come. These benefits may in fact be way better than those in other fields, so it will most likely pay off and pay off big time. But to reach those goals, you have to be patient and prepare yourself mentally to not seek immediate gratification. On the contrary, you should expect it to be tough, rough, exhausting, and mentally challenging. That way, when the desire for immediate gratification does hit you, you are not surprised but instead can quickly shift to a state of acceptance. If you prepare now, then you will be better able to deal with these feelings when they do arise.

The truth is, you will feel pain. You *will* cry many times. You *will* doubt yourself 100 times. You *will* lose friends. People *will* dislike you for no reason. You *will* think you're going crazy. And you *will* come close to talking yourself out of it many times. But understand, this is all just a part of the process! Most of us have felt this way. But you already know what the best part is—it'll all be worth it one day. I promise. (In Chapter 8, you will read the story of when I got this pep talk.)

Opportunities

This chapter will likely scare any student about what's to come. Certainly, there are plenty of challenges to face on the journey to becoming a practicing physician. However, remember that there are also loads of opportunities and advantages to look forward to. Here are just a few[9,10]:

- **Income:** Most physicians earn an above-average income, much higher than professionals in almost any other field. Even in the lowest-paid specialty, you will earn more than six figures; in some specialties, you can make seven figures. Yes, you heard that right. You can make millions in your career as a practicing physician. At the very least, you will lead a comfortable life and rarely worry about your finances—unless you're a foolish spender.
- **Working in other fields:** Medical doctors are highly attractive candidates in fields other than medicine. Many work in business, industry, pharmaceuticals, or consulting. Many also combine their clinical work with other business ventures. Having an "MD" behind your name makes a big impact, and you will find many opportunities outside medicine if you seek them.
- **Doing research:** Many will feel inspired to learn how to conduct research. Medical research is a huge and diverse field. Besides giving you the opportunity to contribute to scientific progress, research can also stimulate a curious mind to make novel discoveries.
- **Helping others:** Health is important to most people. You will have the opportunity to not only understand but also address people's health concerns. Your role as a physician will make you incredibly valuable to others, and in return you will feel deep personal satisfaction. Not many fields offer the chance to provide this unique form of support to people, often at their time of greatest need.
- **Stable job market:** Unless something strange happens, there will likely never be a situation where you will have difficulty finding a job as a physician. Sure, you may not get the exact position you want in your preferred city, but you will find a position somewhere. There are many other fields in which the job market is tough even after someone has earned a master's degree or two. With a medical degree, the job market you are entering is stable and growing.
- **No physical labor:** This is specialty dependent. Obviously, if you're a surgeon, interventional cardiologist, or orthopedist, there may be intense physical labor associated with your work. But for most nonsurgical specialties, you will be doing the mentally hard work of puzzling over diagnoses and how to manage diseases.

These are just a few of the many advantages of being a medical doctor. You are entering a highly sought-after profession. You will be in high demand, and there will be many prospects for you and your career. Therefore, do not let the coming challenges scare you. I have mentioned them to prepare you for what's ahead, because the more prepared you are, the better you will perform. And remember that most people who get into medical school are able to finish it successfully. Rest assured: if they can do it, so can you.

Summary

- Studying in medical school is different than studying in other fields. It has its own set of challenges.
- The medical field combines deep theoretical knowledge with practical knowledge.
- The biggest challenges are the many exams, the multitasking with lecture and practical rotations, the need to learn a lot in a short time, the delayed gratification, and the fact that you will have less of a personal life.

- Being a medical doctor also offers many benefits and opportunities: a high income, a great job market, the ability to help others, the chance to work in fields other than medicine, and the opportunity to contribute to science.
- Going through medical school is a major investment, but one that will pay off. If you work hard for it, you will most likely do well.

References

1. Mitchell CM, Epstein-Peterson ZD, Bandini J, et al. Developing a medical school curriculum for psychological, moral, and spiritual wellness: student and faculty perspectives. *J Pain Symptom Manage.* 2016;52(5):727–736.
2. Reis S. Curriculum reform: Why? What? How? And how will we know it works? *Isr J Health Policy Res.* 2018;7(1):30.
3. Denny JC, Smithers JD, Miller RA, Spickard A 3rd. "Understanding" medical school curriculum content using KnowledgeMap. *J Am Med Inform Assoc.* 2003;10(4):351–362.
4. Raymond JR Sr, Kerschner JE, Hueston WJ, Maurana CA. The merits and challenges of three-year medical school curricula: time for an evidence-based discussion. *Acad Med.* 2015;90(10):1318–1323.
5. Krupat E, Dienstag JL, Kester WC, Finkelstein SN. Medical students who pursue a joint MD/MBA degree: who are they and where are they heading? *Eval Health Prof.* 2017;40(2):203–218.
6. Augustin M. How to learn effectively in medical school: test yourself, learn actively, and repeat in intervals. *Yale J Biol Med.* 2014;87(2):207–212.
7. O'Shea C. Opportunity cost. *Aust Fam Physician.* 2011;40(5):261.
8. Hoerger M, Quirk SW, Weed NC. Development and validation of the Delaying Gratification Inventory. *Psychol Assess.* 2011;23(3):725–738.
9. Owens B. Work-life advantages of becoming a salaried physician may be oversold. *CMAJ.* 2019;191(4):E113–E114. https://doi.org/10.1503/cmaj.109-5699.
10. Zavlin D, Jubbal KT, Noé JG, Gansbacher B. A comparison of medical education in Germany and the United States: from applying to medical school to the beginnings of residency. *Ger Med Sci.* 2017;15: Doc15.

CHAPTER 3

Health Care Literacy

If you can't explain it simply, you don't understand it well enough.
—Albert Einstein

Health literacy is fundamental to quality care.
—Dr. David A. Kindig

Introduction

As a future health care provider, you will play an important role in fostering your patients' health care literacy. Health care literacy is the ability to obtain, process, and understand health information and the services needed to make appropriate health decisions. Health care literacy depends on multiple factors, such as one's knowledge of the area, communication skills, and context of the situation. Recent research shows that the health care information available today is too difficult for the average American to use for making health care decisions[1]. As you begin your medical studies, you will need to digest an enormous amount of information and a huge number of concepts. You should therefore understand what health care literacy is and how you can manage and process all this material in the best way possible.

What is Health Care Literacy?

A person's health care literacy depends on many factors: their cognitive and social skills, the context of what is being discussed, communication skills, and the background of the person who is talking, among other things. The health care situation could involve calculating someone's cholesterol; determining a revised cardiac score index and interpreting the result; measuring medication dosing; or choosing between health insurance plans. As you see, each of these things is totally different and requires different proficiencies.

Health care literacy also requires knowledge of different topics within medicine, which is the most relevant factor for your situation as a medical student. Limited knowledge or misinformation about the body as well as the etiology of disease often causes poor health care literacy—it ultimately leads to a lack of understanding of the relationship between the data in front of you and how to analyze and interpret those data. As stated in the first chapter, to succeed in medical school and as a physician, you need accurate, in-depth knowledge about human biology as well as a clear understanding about why disease happens. You need to know the language of medicine. Moreover, you need to get used to using the language in an accurate way.

In your case, it's all about learning medicine fully and accurately. However, there are so many resources out there that you can get confused and frustrated because you don't know where to start or what to read. The Internet alone has a jungle of information that is easily accessible but not always reliable. Moreover, there is a ton of information out there in general, and you need to be able to read through it and understand it fast. Thus, you need to not only know when to read, but also what to read, how to read, and where to read it.

Hidden Barriers to Understanding and Processing Basic Health Information

Students arrive at medical school with different levels of education and literacy. They come from different cultures and countries. They have different social skills, communication styles, and English language proficiency. All these differences can be barriers to their understanding and teaching of health care information to their future patients.

In medical school, you will have professors and teachers from different backgrounds who have different ways of teaching, which is one of the reasons why you will think some are better teachers than others. Thus, teaching and processing health care information is highly variable depending on who is doing it, where they come from, what language they speak, who taught them, their basic understanding, and so on.

You can never tell whether someone's literacy is good or not just by looking at them. Even if they present themselves well, it does not always mean that they truly know everything in a satisfactory way, nor whether they can present the information in a good way. Some people are merely good presenters. You have to understand that medicine is complex and even the very well educated may still struggle with health-related information[2]. If you see signs of teachers or instructors that are more difficult to understand, do not get nervous or stressed out. There are other resources where you can find information on the topic presented (e.g., textbooks, online articles, and asking other teachers or mentors; see Chapter 9).

Common Health Care Literacy Resources for Medical Students

The Internet has more information than anyone can read in a lifetime or even several lifetimes. But not every website or source of information is reliable. Below is a list of the most common and reliable sources of health care information.

CLASSES

Going to class is one of the best resources for your learning. Even though we have a variety of professors with different educational, language, and health care literacy backgrounds, it is still wise to attend all classes. In the classroom, your teacher will be presenting all the necessary information that you need to know for your learning and also for your exams. It's like going to a restaurant where the meal is served to you instead of cooking the ingredients from scratch at home. The trade-off here is time. You will give up your time to go to class instead of sitting at home and reading. However, if you go to class, you will know what parts of the course are most important and what parts you do not need to focus on. However, classes are not for everyone. Some students do not function best by listening to someone lecture—they learn better by reading on their own. There could be many reasons for their preference: the speed of the presenter, the presentation itself, health care literacy, individual learning abilities, and so on[3]. It is reasonable to read by yourself at home as long as you use the time well and read accurately instead of doing other things.

TEXTBOOKS—PRINT BOOKS AND EBOOKS

Medical textbooks are by far the primary source of the knowledge you will get in medical school. Either experts in the field or knowledgeable and experienced physicians have typically written these textbooks. Most of them are also referenced, which means that each statement you read is backed up by science. Therefore, books should be your focus after your lectures. However, these textbooks could be hundreds or thousands of pages long, which makes it difficult to grasp and remember everything. This is why guidance from your classes and professors is so important—it will allow you to filter what is high yield and what is not[4]. Also, this guide will tell you more about how to strategically read, understand, and remember a large amount of information (see Chapter 7).

MEDICAL JOURNALS

Today, there are thousands of medical journals published, on every topic imaginable. Many of these journals publish legitimate manuscripts, while others do not. What makes a medical journal a good one depends on many factors, but the main reasons are their credibility, their impact factor (IF), how many times they are cited, and their peer-review process. The higher the IF, the greater the credibility, and the more rigorous the peer-review process, the better the journal[5]. High IF journals are more selective about the papers they accept and therefore more desirable to authors. The IF is a measure of the frequency with which the average article in a journal has been cited in a particular year. It is often used to assess the rank and importance of a journal[6]. For instance, the top medical journals in the world based on their IF are *The New England Journal of Medicine*, *Nature*, *The Lancet*, *Science*, and *The Journal of the American Medical Association* (JAMA).

Whenever a manuscript is submitted to a journal, it undergoes peer review, which means that experts read and analyze the paper and determine its impact, usefulness, reliability, relevance, and methods used to conduct the study. The harder the peer-review process, the more difficult it is to get a paper accepted to a journal. A journal with a rigorous peer-review process is more selective and therefore will only accept high-quality manuscripts. For example, *The New England Journal of Medicine* is considered one of the top medical journals in the world. It receives thousands of manuscripts per year but it only accepts a small percentage of them[7]. Other journals may have a higher acceptance rate, which means that lower-quality papers get accepted as well as manuscripts and research papers that contain errors.

By now you should understand that not every paper that gets published has conclusions that are reliable. Journals with a higher IF and more rigorous review process are those whose articles have been analyzed by experts in the field. In such cases, you can be more assured that the reviewers have a much better idea about the state of the art in that field as well as the knowledge gaps. Therefore, if a paper is accepted for publication in a high IF journal, it is likely that the authors have discovered something genuinely new and meaningful that not even the experts were aware of.

In general, reading high IF journals is a good thing and something that you will be doing in medical school[9]. However, aiming to learn all your medical knowledge from medical journals is not the best strategy. Most recently published articles are on the cutting edge in a particular area. Conversely, early in your medical career, you need to focus on acquiring more general knowledge about the area as a whole. Furthermore, searching through medical journals on a specific topic could be useful but typically takes time you don't have, and you may not even get all the information you need in the end. Therefore, medical journals should be used whenever they are assigned to you by your professor or if you need to dig deeper into a topic. For instance, there are review papers and other informative manuscripts that might have the information you need. But stick to reading papers from high IF journals to ensure you are getting reliable information. Otherwise, it will be time consuming and low yield. In summary, as a medical student, you can use medical journals as a supplement to your textbooks but don't make them your primary source of knowledge.

FORUMS

Again, just as there are thousands of medical journals, there are countless medical forums online. Many of these are created by physicians and medical students based in the United States and abroad. The advantage of these forums is that you have access to fellow students at your level or above with whom you can discuss any topic. The forums often keep archives of past posts. Thus it is likely that if you search the forum, you will find that your question has already been answered. You might want to consider becoming a member of some of the more popular forums as a way to enhance your learning. But remember, the information presented may not always be reliable depending on who has written it. So proceed with caution and always confirm the accuracy of the information stated. Forums should guide you in the right direction and are good sources to quickly look up basic facts, but these should always be confirmed with textbooks to ensure that the knowledge is accurate[8].

WIKIPEDIA AND OTHER WEBSITES

Wikipedia is an example of a website that covers many medical topics. However, just about anybody, including those without a medical background, can and does write for Wikipedia, which means that one cannot always trust the content. There are also other sites written by medical students or journalists that could very well have the correct information at times, but might also at other times be wrong. Processing and rewriting medical information is not always easy, and there are many things that could be misunderstood, especially when you don't have a medical degree. Consequently, to make sure you are obtaining the right information from the start, you should avoid websites like Wikipedia except as an adjunct to more reliable sources of information.

Practical Strategies

In medical school, you will find yourself in lectures where you won't understand a thing. Conversely, you will also find yourself in classes where you will grasp most of the information. Don't panic! This is common and something that all medical students struggle with. You always have your books to fall back on. The most important advice here is to take notes about the different topics that your lecturer is presenting on, write down as much as you can about them, and then read about the topics later in your book or ask your classmates about things you don't understand. Certain topics will be complicated no matter how good the presenter is at explaining. For instance, understanding the different anatomic locations of a specific bone is very different from understanding DNA replication.

Summary

- Health care literacy is the ability to obtain, process, and understand health information and the services needed to make appropriate health decisions.
- Students arrive at medical school with different levels of education and literacy. They come from different cultures and countries. They have different social skills, communication styles, and English language proficiency. All these differences can be barriers to their understanding and teaching of health care information to their future patients.
- In medical school, you will have professors and teachers from different backgrounds who have different ways of teaching, which is one of the reasons why you will think some are better teachers than others.
- Learn from reliable sources. Do not trust all sources online, and do not waste your time on researchers that will not give you a high return on your investment of time. Some sources are not backed up by science, and some are too cutting edge.
- Classes and lectures are recommended to attend, since your teacher will be presenting the necessary information that you need to know for your learning and also for your exams.
- By far, medical textbooks are your best source of information for studying, as they contain the core knowledge that you will be learning in medical school.

References

1. Office of Disease Prevention and Health Promotion. Health Literacy. Health.gov. https://health.gov/our-work/health-literacy. Updated February 5, 2020. Accessed September 16, 2020.
2. Davis T. Agency for Healthcare Research and Quality. Healthcare Literacy: Hidden Barriers and Practical Strategies. https://www.ahrq.gov/professionals/quality-patient-safety/quality-resources/tools/literacy-toolkit/tool3a/index.html. Published January 2015. Updated December 2017. Accessed September 16, 2020.
3. Murphy B. American Medical Association. Why Some Medical Students Are Cutting Class to Get Ahead. https://www.ama-assn.org/residents-students/medical-school-life/why-some-medical-students-are-cutting-class-get-ahead. Published February 4, 2019. Accessed September 16, 2020.
4. Gupta M. Stanford Medicine. You Are What You Read: The Academic Diet of the 21st-Century Medical Student. https://scopeblog.stanford.edu/2014/01/22/you-are-what-you-read-the-academic-diet-of-the-21st-century-medical-student/. Published January 22, 2014. Accessed September 16, 2020.
5. Wikipedia. Wikipedia.org. https://en.wikipedia.org/wiki/Wikipedia. Accessed September 16, 2020.
6. Menon D. The World's Top Medical Journals—A Guide. Health Writer Hub. https://www.healthwriter-hub.com/top-medical-journals. Published April 21, 2015. Updated July 9, 2019. Accessed September 16, 2020.
7. University Library, University of Illinois-Chicago. Measuring Your Impact: Impact Factor, Citation Analysis, and Other Metrics: Journal Impact Factor (IF). https://researchguides.uic.edu/if/impact. Updated February 8, 2020. Accessed September 16, 2020.
8. John M. The target journal: choosing the right place to submit your paper. *HSR Proc Intensive Care Cardiovasc Anesth.* 2009;1(3):60–62.
9. Slinn K. Is 'High-Yield' Learning Making Future Docs Less Prepared? Medscape.com. https://www.medscape.com/viewarticle/910353. Published March 18, 2019.

CHAPTER 4

Motivation and Mindset

The harder you work for something, the greater you'll feel when you achieve it.
—Unknown

Once your mindset changes, everything on the outside will change along with it.
—Steve Maraboli

The Physiology Behind Motivation

Learning about motivation is important to succeed in life. It's especially important where you are concerned, as medicine is one of the toughest programs there is.

"Motivation" has many definitions, but the one that I like best is this one: motivation is "the reasons you have for doing, acting or behaving in a particular way"[1]. But what does this mean? Have you ever asked yourself what motivation really means? Why are you motivated to eat things that you like, while you are not motivated to eat things you dislike? Why are you motivated to watch TV shows that you enjoy? Why are you motivated to do the activities you do as opposed to doing other things? Why, for instance, are you not always motivated to get out of bed at five in the morning? Why are you not always motivated to go to school, sit in class all day, and then come home to study? These are important questions to ask so that you can find out what motivation really is.

The answer is simple: You are motivated to do things that reward you and make you feel good. When you eat a chocolate bar, the reward is the taste of the chocolate. When you watch your favorite TV show, your reward is the entertainment it gives to your brain, whether it's joy, happiness, or perhaps inspiration. When you hang out with your friends, you receive the social reward of friendship. In short, we feel motivated to do things that provide us with *mental or physical rewards*[2,3].

So why isn't school motivating then? Why is it still so hard to get up in the morning and go to school? Why is it so hard to sit down and study for hours? There are two main reasons for this: one, you may not understand or acknowledged the true reward or benefit of your education yet,

19

and two, because getting up and studying is not giving you an *instant* reward, such as when you eat a chocolate bar or watch TV.

For the most part, the painful truth is that studying in school will never give you the instant joy and satisfaction that you get from many other entertaining and enjoyable things (like chocolate, TV, and your friends). That is why this entire chapter is dedicated to making you understand what motivation is, why it is important, and how studying hard in medical school can reward you—perhaps not in the short term, but most definitely in the long term. Once you understand the purpose and benefits of studying hard now, you will be motivated to do so *and* to do it well.

Without motivation, it is hard to succeed in anything. This is why this topic is extremely important and deserves its own chapter. It won't matter how much you study or how much time you spend in school if you feel unmotivated. All that work will prove to be exhausting, and you will fail in some way in the long run. Without the proper motivation, the experience of medical school will end up being frustrating and hard. If you are not motivated, it could mean that you spend hours and hours studying without getting good results. School will be meaningless if you do not find the motivation to do it right[2,3].

Extrinsic Versus Intrinsic Motivation

Extrinsic motivation is when you perform or do something to earn a reward or avoid punishment, not because you enjoy it or because you find it satisfying, but in order to get something in return or to avoid something unpleasant (Figure 4.1). A classic example of extrinsic motivation is when a professor sets a deadline on a research project and the bonus is tied to that deadline[4].

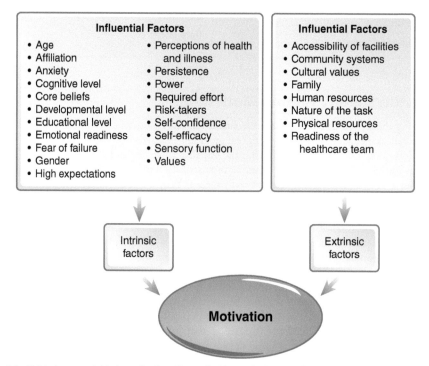

Fig. 4.1 Extrinsic versus intrinsic motivation. (Reused with permission from Giddens JF. *Concepts for Nursing Practice.* Elsevier; 2013. Figure 5-2, Relationships Between Intrinsic and Extrinsic Factors and Motivation.)

Intrinsic motivation, on the other hand, is when you do something that is personally rewarding (see Figure 4.1). You are engaging in a behavior for *yourself* or for its own sake rather than the desire for some external reward[4]. This motivation arrives from *within*, compared with extrinsic motivation, which arrives from the outside. You strive towards a goal for personal satisfaction or accomplishment. The motivation is internal. Which one do you think is better?

Many studies have shown that intrinsic motivation is superior to extrinsic motivation when it comes to learning, getting good grades, and succeeding in school[6-8]. There is a proverb that goes "You can lead a horse to water, but you can't make it drink." In fact, extrinsic rewards do not lead to intrinsic motivation or long-term change. By contrast, extrinsic rewards reduce intrinsic motivation and the desire to try. Meaningful work, such as studying medicine and becoming a good doctor, must be driven by intrinsic rather than extrinsic motivation. This is also why it's often said that you should "do things for the right reasons."

Many people can find temporary external motivation, such as by watching an inspirational video or reading a motivational quote. These are all good, but only temporary. It is far more important to find inner motivation so that you will feel motivated every single day. Whenever you want to achieve a big dream, you must harness this inner motivation in order to follow through on the hard work of getting there. This motivation will then serve as energy for your body, just like fuel for a car, and will push you forward so that you do not stagnate. Once you have the motivation for doing difficult things, you are more likely to want to do them, do them well, and get continuously better at doing them. Everything gets easier and goes much faster. Motivation becomes your driving force, the inner voice that keeps telling you to get up at five in the morning even though it's cold, dark, and windy outside and you are very, very tired.

Value Creation

So how do you get motivated to do something you don't want to do? It requires two things:
1. Set meaningful long-term goals and see the goals as your reward, and
2. Measure the value of your rewards.

Setting goals is relatively straightforward to understand; you will learn how to do this in Chapter 5. A meaningful goal is one that will give you your preferred reward in the end. Whether that goal is to be a surgeon or travel around the world, these goals will give you the joy of doing what you want to do or experience. Seeing the value of the rewards is usually what students have a hard time with.

There are very few people on the planet who would rather wake up early in the morning, go to class all day, then come home to study all night until it's time for bed, day in and day out, when instead they could be out with friends, shopping, playing video games, or watching TV. Both of these paths give you rewards in the end, but the important difference is that only one of these paths offers you enormous value in the future.

Let me give you an example. If your dad asks you to throw out the trash on a Saturday evening in the middle of winter, and you know you have to walk 500 feet to get to the trash can, you will probably not feel a strong motivation to do so. You will walk with heavy, frustrating steps with the trash bag in your hands and will not care if there is a lot of junk pouring out from the bags. You will likely be busy thinking, "I hate doing this." You will not do a good job. In fact, the entire effort will be frustrating for you. Why? Because you do not *want to* do it. You feel no motivation to throw out the trash. You don't see the reward of doing so. You don't see the value. When you think that you are forced to do something that does not favor or reward you, you will never perform well. You would never think that throwing out the trash would favor or reward you. In fact, throwing out the trash does you more good than staying in bed and watching TV. But you don't see it like that. You don't see the reward in it. Why? Because the reward is not an *instant reward*. It does not give you instant joy.

The fact of delayed rewards is one of the most fundamental things for you to understand. Throwing out the trash is not like eating good chocolate and instantly savoring its deliciousness in your mouth. It's not like playing video games where your brain gets constant jolts of excitement. But, if you think twice about it, throwing out the garbage instead of lying in your bed watching TV has more rewards and value than you realize. You are contributing to a more sanitary environment at home; you are helping your dad; you are standing up and walking, which is healthier than lying down. The issue is that we don't see or appreciate these kinds of rewards when they are not accompanied by instant pleasure.

This is the exact same issue that many students have with school. You may not see or derive instant benefits or rewards by studying day in and day out, going to class, staying focused, doing your best on your medical rotations, and so on. You therefore don't find the motivation for doing it. The result is that you will not invest the necessary time in doing it well. However, once you learn to see the rewards of working hard in school and then evaluating the value of things, you will change your priorities and find the inner motivation you need.

The fact is that medical school provides you with far more value and rewards than most other things do. At least at your age. But this is a long-term reward, not an instant one. It will not give you several million dollars tomorrow, but it could earn you that much money in 10 to 20 years. So, you have to learn to distinguish between short- and long-term rewards, and you have to learn to assess the value of the much smaller rewards that your daily actions yield.

Will talking on the phone with your friends, going out to party every night, and watching TV when you get home from school give you your dream life in the future? Probably not. But will studying hard in school, doing well on your tests, getting good grades, and matching into your desired specialty give you a good life? That's much more likely! Watching TV will give you the instant reward of joy that reading an anatomy book won't. But reading the anatomy book will give you much more value in life for your purpose than if you watched TV, and a much higher reward in the long run. So the concept is easy. Every day when you wake up, you should think about the things that will give you the biggest reward and the highest value in life. The key is to see the long-term rewards and values of every action you take. Sure, partying, hanging out, and watching TV are all fun, but how much long-term value will they bring to your future life? Not much. If you choose those low-value activities today and every day after that, then you are essentially throwing away your dream of becoming a doctor in your desired specialty.

Exams, homework, assignments, and endless hours of studying may seem like a burden to you right now because you will not get those instant rewards that you're accustomed to getting from other easy things. But if I flip the question and ask you, Do you want to be successful in your medical career, become a great doctor in your desired field, and get a good job that you enjoy with a high salary that gives you opportunities in life? I bet the answer to that is yes. If so, then you understand that spending time on low-value activities won't give you that life. Putting in the time to learn physiology, pharmacology, and anatomy will give you the knowledge to do well on your tests, which will lead to good grades. In turn, you will finish medical school more successfully and be a more competitive applicant in the residency match process. And when you do finish medical school, you will have the best opportunities to do whatever it is you want to do. At this stage of your life, there is likely nothing that will bring you more value than studying and finishing medical school with the best grades, knowledge, and credentials. And once you adopt this mindset, you will be intrinsically motivated to work hard in school.

Creating Motivation

So, to get intrinsically motivated, you need to set your goals and assess your values:

1. Set your goals:
   - What are your goals for your medical career?

- What specialty do you see yourself in?
- What do you want to achieve as a doctor?
- Where would you like to work?
- Who would you like to serve?

These goals are your rewards because they are your biggest dreams. And the bigger the dreams, the better. Write down your goals.

2. Assess your values:
- Identify the value of your daily actions in life.
- What actions can you perform every day to give you the most long-term benefit?

The things that will bring you the highest value, the best return? Those are the things you have to do every day. And obviously, the answer at this stage of your life is that you need to put the most time and energy into finishing your homework; preparing for your tests, exams, and rotations; and getting the best grades and scores possible so that you can feel intrinsically motivated to achieve your goals and dreams (step 1).

You will now be motivated to do things that you didn't want to do before. Why? Because now you understand motivation and see the value in things that don't bring instant rewards. You see the value of doing things that will bring you closer to your dreams—your biggest long-term rewards in life[7,8].

Motivate Yourself With the Following Thought Process

What is the reward of being a good student and working hard in school? Good grades, matching into an exciting and competitive specialty, graduating from the best residency training programs, getting a great job with a high salary, and having a great future. You are free to do whatever you want: travel the world, meet your material needs, start a business, do good for society, and so much more.

Remember that from this day forward, don't let yourself be fooled into doing things that are guaranteed to give you instant rewards. Most of these instant rewards will waste your time and prevent you from reaching your goals and achieving your dreams. Sure, we all need a break from time to time, and that's okay, but don't let the breaks get out of hand. Breaks should be short and useful, meaning they should only take a fraction of your time and reenergize your brain for those high-value activities.

Summary

- Motivation is the reasons you have for acting or behaving in a particular way. Without motivation, it is hard to succeed in anything.
- Extrinsic motivation is when you perform or do something to earn a reward or avoid punishment, not because you enjoy it or because you find it satisfying.
- Intrinsic motivation is when you do something that is personally rewarding. The motivation comes from within.
- Intrinsic motivation is far superior to extrinsic motivation, since meaningful work such as becoming a good doctor is driven by intrinsic rather than extrinsic factors.
- Intrinsic motivation comes from (1) setting meaningful long-term goals and seeing the goals as your reward and (2) measuring the value of your rewards and seeing the value in your daily actions.
- The greatest benefit comes from doing the high-value activities that help you achieve your long-term dream of becoming a physician in your chosen specialty. Anything that doesn't contribute to your dreams and goals is a low-value activity and should be avoided.

References

1. Motivation. Google Dictionary. https://google.com/. Accessed September 16, 2020.
2. Mahler D, Großschedl J, Harms U. Does motivation matter? The relationship between teachers' self-efficacy and enthusiasm and students' performance. *PLoS One.* 2018;13(11):e0207252.
3. Cook DA, Artino AR Jr. Motivation to learn: an overview of contemporary theories. *Med Educ.* 2016;50(10):997–1014.
4. Ramirez-Andreotta MD, Tapper A, Clough D, Carrera JS, Sandhaus S. Understanding the intrinsic and extrinsic motivations associated with community gardening to improve environmental public health prevention and intervention. *Int J Environ Res Public Health.* 2019;16(3):494. https://doi.org/10.3390/ijerph16030494.
5. Lee W, Reeve J, Xue Y, Xiong J. Neural differences between intrinsic reasons for doing versus extrinsic reasons for doing: an fMRI study. *Neurosci Res.* 2012;73(1):68–72. https://doi.org/10.1016/j.neures.2012.02.010.
6. Di Domenico SI, Ryan RM. The emerging neuroscience of intrinsic motivation: a new frontier in self-determination research. *Front Hum Neurosci.* 2017;11:145. https://doi.org/10.3389/fnhum.2017.00145.
7. Roberts H. Creating motivation, identifying incentives and enablers, and encouraging staff development. *Community Eye Health.* 2005;18(56):122–124.
8. Preziosi RC. Ten ways to create a motivating learning environment. *Hosp Mater Manage Q.* 1995;17(2):53–58.

CHAPTER 5

Goals and Goal Setting

All successful people have a goal. No one can get anywhere unless he knows where he wants to go and what he wants to be or do.
—Norman Vincent Peale

All who have accomplished great things have had a great aim, have fixed their gaze on a goal which was high, one which sometimes seemed impossible.
—Orison Swett Marden

You have to set goals that are almost out of reach. If you set a goal that is attainable without much work or thought, you are stuck with something below your true talent and potential.
—Steve Garvey

What is a Goal?

Goals are extremely powerful. Every person should set goals in their lives at all times. It is one of the few things that pushes us forward in life and makes us achieve incredible things. A goal can be defined as a desired result, envisioned by you, which then is accompanied by an effort aimed at achieving it[1]. For centuries, successful people have known the power of setting goals. Much of what exists around us in modern cities was made possible because of people like you and me who had goals. The phone in your hand, the car that you drive, the medications that you take—they are all inventions dreamed up by people who had a vision and goal.

If you asked someone 100 years ago whether it would have been possible to one day land on the moon, most people would have probably laughed at you and called you crazy. Back then, it was unthinkable that someone could build a spacecraft capable of landing on the moon. Today, we have not only been to the moon, but we are sending spacecrafts to other planets. Many accomplishments that were once considered impossible are now a reality, and this trend will continue in the future as well. Things *become* possible because we set goals and have a vision. Without goals or a vision, nothing much ever happens. But equipped with clear goals and a vision, we can somehow always come up with solutions to problems standing in the way of our dreams, no matter how hard and bumpy the road. That is how the mind works. But first, you need to see it in your head, and that "seeing" process is the actual goal setting itself.

What people with nearly impossible dreams also understood was that they had to divide their big goal (landing on the moon, for instance) into smaller milestones. In the case of the moon landing, scientists had to figure out, among other things, the distance to the moon, the environment in space, the resources needed to get there, how to train astronauts, how to build a spacecraft, and so on. Finally, on July 20, 1969, Apollo 11 landed on the moon, and Neil Armstrong became the first human to ever set foot on the moon's surface[2].

As with the moon landing, in order to achieve *your* big goals, you first have to divide them into smaller subgoals or milestones. Each of your milestones will require plenty of hard work and preparation. Your daily efforts will gradually snowball into the eventual achievement of your bigger goal. The completion of your individual milestones requires a structured approach that is taken one day at a time. First, you need to devise a plan and a strategy to reach your milestones. You can't just press a button and, voilà, be teleported to the future. You have to set goals, divide them into smaller goals, and then plan and work toward them so that all the great things you want to achieve in life actually happen. And if you do that, you'll be unstoppable[3].

Why Are Goals Important?

Any successful person can tell you about the power of goal setting. Setting goals is not just an exercise you do in your head or words you scribble on a piece of paper, to be forgotten in a drawer. Goal setting involves chemical reactions in your brain. Something "magical" literally happens when you set goals the right way. You start the process of moving toward the dreams you want to achieve. Your brain starts to process thoughts and ideas on how to get there. Your unconscious pulls you toward your goal, and your mental antenna starts to register everything that is needed to take you there. Setting goals is one of the not-so-secret secrets to succeeding in medical school and in life[3,4].

Goals give your reasons, your "why," your purpose. Reasons to start doing things. Reasons to get up in the morning, go to school, learn the course material the best you can, and get those good grades. If you have enough reasons to start acting upon your goals, you will do things you never thought possible. If you have enough purpose in your life, you will develop the routines needed to become successful. And these reasons will change your whole life.

Many students have high intelligence and plenty of resources and abilities. But what they lack is reasons and goals. I personally think that your current grades may not reflect your true intelligence. Unless you have always been a straight A student, I think you're actually much smarter than what your current educational performance indicates. So why are you not doing better? Why are your grades not better? Most likely because you don't have enough goals and reasons. Reasons come first. Results come second. You will not do well until you have reasons for doing well. Once you have reasons, the answers to how you do things or achieve things will come more easily. Goals give you reasons, and reasons will give you the intrinsic motivation and energy to do the things necessary to reach your goals. Consequently, you will start seeing much better results[3,4].

The Types of Goals to Set in Medical School

Let us look at some of the goals that are important to have in medical school.
   1. **Personal reasons.** Some people do it for themselves. They set up goals to excel. To become the best medical student or doctor possible. The best physician a patient can meet. They

do it for the recognition and respect. They love the feeling of being a winner and getting better. Those are good reasons. I have doctor friends who are already making extremely high salaries, but they keep working 10 to 12 hours a day to make millions more. Not because they need the money, but because they want the enjoyment and satisfaction of being a winner, an outstanding physician. As a result, some people do things, including working hard for good grades, for personal satisfaction.

2. **Desired specialty.** Some specialties in medicine are highly competitive. Only the best students match into them. Examples of these specialties are plastic surgery, dermatology, and neurosurgery. In order to match into these specialties and complete the residency training, you need to be a straight-A student, ace your school exams and the United States Medical Licensing Examination (USMLE), and excel on your rotations. This level of achievement requires goal setting. To achieve a certain score on the USMLE, you need to set a goal. To excel on your rotations, you also need to set certain goals.

3. **Personal development.** Some people do it simply to learn more and become more knowledgeable. They are lifelong students. They want to expand their knowledge base.

Goal setting is important not just in life, but also as part of your path to becoming a successful medical doctor.

When students enter medical school, they often don't have a specific goal in mind about what specialty to choose upon graduation. Most want to go through different rotations first so they can see what fits them best. This is absolutely fine. However, what often ends up happening is that some students do not understand that certain specialties are highly competitive. Their academic performance isn't as good as it can be. And by the time they have made up their minds, it's too late. So they end up choosing a field based not on their interests but rather on what their grades and other achievements are in line with. To me, that is the wrong approach.

Unlike others, when I started medical school, I knew what I wanted to do. But even if I didn't, my strategy was always to perform as well as possible in each and every situation so that I could choose whatever specialty I wanted later on. Therefore, even if you do not know what you want to do after medical school, I suggest that you set goals to achieve the best possible outcome each year so that you can choose a specialty according to your personal preferences and interests later on.

You might be curious about what an ideal candidate looks like for those highly competitive specialties such as plastic surgery, dermatology, and neurosurgery. Many would agree on the following criteria[5]:

- Graduated at the top of your class
- Achieved excellent USMLE Step 1 and Step 2 scores
- Member of the Alpha Omega Alpha Honor Society
- Published numerous papers
- Demonstrates maturity
- Exhibits leadership qualities
- Respected by your peers
- Have excellent letters of recommendations from known people in the field, and
- Have done well on your rotations.

Even if you are not looking to matching into a competitive specialty, this list of accomplishments is something that you should try to achieve regardless. You'll want to reach these goals not just to be able to match into whatever specialty you want later on, but also for personal reasons. If you fit many of the above criteria, you will most likely also develop profound knowledge in the medical field, be a great and respected medical student, and have a high level of personal development.

How to Set Goals

Now you know that goals are important. You know why they are important, and you also have insight in what type of goals to set when you start medical school. We can therefore finally get into how to set your goals, which is the final important step[6,7].

1. **Define your goals.** The first step is to define your big goals. Sit down and really think about it. Goal setting is not something that takes just a few minutes. It requires active engagement of your imagination. Sit down and thoroughly think about what your goals are for medical school. Why did you want to become a doctor? Was it for the passion? Interest? Money? A good lifestyle? A comfortable life? Whatever your reasons are, they should be well thought out. Define your big goal by thinking carefully about what *you* want in life. Do not bother about what others want or what they intend to do. You are your own person and have individual needs that you want to satisfy in your life. Just because some people want to do certain things does not mean that their path will be the best path for you. Never forget that, and never let anyone unduly influence your vision. Take your time here. Sometimes, it can take many sessions, days, or weeks before you know what your true goals are.

2. **Ask yourself why.** The next step is to think about *why* you want to achieve these goals. This step is incredibly important because it gives your goals meaning. Many people say that they want to make a lot of money, but when you dig further and ask them why, they don't have a good answer other than saying that they could buy nice things—but that's not a meaningful reason. A genuine goal has a deeper purpose behind it. If you really want to achieve something, you should have at least one or several reasons for wanting it. Think about why you want to achieve your big goals.

3. **Write down your goals.** No matter what you do, don't keep your goals in your head. You will forget them. Write them down. And the more detail you include, the better. Two things happen when you write down goals: external storage and encoding. Here is why that is important:

   - *External storage* means that you are storing the information, usually on a piece of paper, that you can access and review any time. This process makes you look at your goal many times, remember it, and constantly think about. And the more you think about something, the more magnetically you will be drawn to it. The opposite is a known phenomenon: when we do not think or pay attention to something for a long time, we tend to forget about it. Out of sight, out of mind.

   - Encoding is the deeper process. This is a biological process whereby your goal is transferred to the memory area of your brain and then analyzed. Here, the brain makes decisions about what to store in short-term versus long-term memory. Writing down your goals improves the encoding process. Consequently, this makes you remember your goal much better. Again, the more you remember your goals, the better your focus and energy, and the better your chance of achieving your goals.

4. **Establish your milestones.** Once your big goals are defined, the real hard work begins. At this stage, you should divide your big goals into smaller milestones, and then further divide those milestones into even smaller subgoals. For example, building a rocket was one of the milestones for getting to the moon. But building a rocket also needed to be divided into smaller subgoals in order to be achieved. To divide your big goals into smaller milestones and subgoals, identify the exact steps that are required to make your big goal a reality. Write down exactly what steps must be taken and how these should be organized. That is, step 1, step 2, step 3, and so on. In this way, you will set up action steps with smaller milestones that will lead you to reaching your big goal.

5. **List your action steps.** Once you've set up your milestones and smaller goals, it's time to develop a plan. This is your strategy or action steps. Develop a to-do list of things that needs to be accomplished in order to achieve your goals. Simply writing down your goals on paper is not enough. You also need to have a plan and work toward that plan to make it a reality.

6. **Determine your time frame.** Each goal needs to have a realistic timeline attached to it. It would be great if we had 20 years to achieve each goal. This is an example of an unrealistic time frame. Setting a time frame for each of your milestones, subgoals, and to-do items will create a sense of urgency that will motivate you toward reaching your goals at a faster pace.

7. **Stick with it.** Once you have set up your big goals, milestones, smaller subgoals, action steps, a strategy and plan, and a time frame, you have to stick with your goals. This part is so important. Remember that the goals you've written down are the things you really want in your life, and many of them are not going to be easy to accomplish. But they are not impossible either. Human beings have done so many unique, creative, and seemingly impossible things in our history on this planet. If people once did such difficult things, you can too. But only those who stuck with their plans regardless of how tough it got are the ones who succeeded in the end. If you want to reach your goals bad enough, you will find a way to do it if you don't give up.

Here is an example of how set up and organize a goal:

- **Big goal:** Get into a dermatologist residency.
- **Why:** I have a huge interest in skin disorders; I prioritize lifestyle; my research is in the field of skin disorders.
- **Milestones:** Graduate top of my class; do very well on USMLE Step 1 and Step 2; publish extensively within dermatology; network with big names in dermatology; present papers at dermatology meetings; become an Alpha Omega Alpha Honor Society member.
- **Smaller milestones/subgoals:** Do very well on every rotation in medical school; get top scores on my medical school exams; study strategically and hard for the USMLEs; do dermatology rotations at well-known institutions and participate in their research.
- **Plan/strategy:** Ask other successful medical students how they excelled in their rotations; ask and actively do research on how to ace the medical school exams; build a strategy on how to study for the exams and USMLEs; set up a daily, weekly, and monthly plan for studying.
- **Time frame:**
  - Dermatology residency: 4 years
  - Graduate top of my class: 4 years
  - Do well on USMLE Step 1: 1 year
  - Do well on USMLE Step 2: 2 years
  - Etc.

As you can see, each goal has multiple milestones or subgoals. To make the plan something you can use to keep yourself on track, the key is to divide each goal into smaller milestones and subgoals. And the smaller and more detailed they are, the better.

Summary

- A goal is a desired result, envisioned by you, which then is accompanied by an effort aimed at achieving it.
- Goals are powerful. They energize you and make you achieve things you want in life.
- There are many type of goals to set in medical school based on personal preference.

■ Goal can be set by following this algorithm: define your goals; ask yourself why; write down your goals; establish your milestones; list your action steps; determine your time frame; and, last but not least, stick with it.

References

1. Goal. Google Dictionary. https://google.com/. Accessed September 16, 2020.
2. July 20, 1969: One Giant Leap For Mankind. NASA.gov. https://www.nasa.gov/mission_pages/apollo/apollo11.html. Updated July 15, 2019. Accessed November 20, 2019.
3. Fuhrmann CN, Hobin JA, Clifford PS, et al. Goal-Setting Strategies for Scientific and Career Success. Sciencemag.org. https://www.sciencemag.org/careers/2013/12/goal-setting-strategies-scientific-and-career-success. Published December 3, 2013.
4. Sadowski E, Schrager S. Achieving career satisfaction: personal goal setting and prioritizing for the clinician educator. *J Grad Med Educ.* 2016;8(4):494–497.
5. Mitsouras K, Dong F, Safaoui MN, Helf SC. Student academic performance factors affecting matching into first-choice residency and competitive specialties. *BMC Med Educ.* 2019;19(1):241. 1.
6. Golden Rules of Goal Setting. MindTools.com. https://www.mindtools.com/pages/article/newHTE_90.htm. Accessed June 2, 2016.
7. Murphy M. Neuroscience Explains Why You Need to Write Down Your Goals If You Actually Want to Achieve Them. Forbes.com. https://www.forbes.com/sites/markmurphy/2018/04/15/neuroscience-explains-why-you-need-to-write-down-your-goals-if-you-actually-want-to-achieve-them/#4863b8fd7905. Published April 15, 2018.

CHAPTER 6

Time Management

Use your time wisely. Time is what we want most, but what we use worst.
Will Penn

Time Management and Its Importance

Your years in medical school years will be busy times. You will have a lot of courses, classes, rotations, homework, assignments, exams, and many other things that you need to complete in a relatively short time. Not only do you need to complete these tasks, you need to complete them well. This is where time management comes into play. Time management is the process of organizing and planning how to divide your time between specific activities, enabling you to work smarter, not harder. It lets you get more things done in less time, which reduces stress and pressure and enables you to perform much better.

You are likely familiar with the common interview question, "Where do you see yourself in 10 years?" The reason why so many interviewers ask this question is that they want to see what the candidate's plan is for the future. It would be a mistake to answer "I don't know" or "I take each day as it comes." Your interviewers will not be impressed with your response, as very few things in life should be unplanned or left to chance. Such an answer shows a lack of thoughtfulness, preparation, and planning on your part.

One of the major factors that will determine your success in anything is creating a plan and a strategy, then making sure you follow them. If you ask any successful person, they will tell you that they indeed have a plan, one that is well organized and structured. They plan out every single project and make sure they follow the plan religiously. Without a plan and an effective way of managing your time, it will be extremely difficult to accomplish your goals and to perform well in medical school.

So how do you manage a busy schedule with multiple things to do in a short time? By having a plan and being good at time management.

Time—Your Most Precious Resource

The better you plan your life, the more you'll get out of it. Do you remember how long days seemed when you were a kid? It felt like you had all the time in the world. You got up in the morning and watched TV, then went to the kitchen and had breakfast. Maybe after that you played in your room for a while, and then you headed to the playground across the street to play with your friends. Sometime later, your parents would call for you to come home for lunch. And after lunch, you *still* had the entire rest of the day to enjoy. Those were the days!

Once we hit adolescence and adulthood, however, it feels as though the days are only getting shorter and shorter and that time is passing faster and faster. I'm probably not alone in sometimes wishing that a day would last 48 hours instead of 24 hours. But that will never be. With only 24 hours in a day, it is essential that you learn to use your time and energy wisely so that you can keep up with everything that is important to your success. The key is to thoughtfully plan your life, your studies, your job, and everything else and to understand how to manage your time. By doing so, you will organize everything and your life will be structured so you know what and when to do things.

Time is your most precious resource in medical school and in life. If you and I had 20 years to finish medical school, we could do things very slowly and perhaps without having a detailed plan. However, this is not the case. This is the reason why you have a schedule in school. When you start your first week in school, you get a schedule that ensures you can finish all the necessary courses for the semester on time and that outlines what you need to learn by the end of each semester[1].

Just like your school schedule, you should make your own life schedule (or plan) so that you can create the structure in your life to carry out your activities wisely. Planning your time is one of the most important factors for achieving top grades in all your courses and rotations. Therefore, from day one, you have to start planning your entire medical education[1].

Why Time Management in Medicine is Different From That in Other Fields

Time management is especially important in medical school because, unlike most programs, you are expected to do a lot in a very short time: you have to go to class, learn the content, take exams, and complete assignments. On top of that, once you start your third year, you will also have clinical rotations—these are critical to your long-term success. You will be evaluated and graded on these rotations. Some of these rotations may eat up a big chunk of your day. Surgical rotations are examples of busy rotations where you sometimes start at five in the morning and will not finish until late afternoon. At the same time, you will have exams too, so you need to study for these simultaneously. Very few programs outside of medicine expose students to such a grueling schedule. It is therefore critical that you have a well-rounded plan so you know when and what to study at all times[2].

Balancing the Hours of the Day

When you look at the 24 hours we all have in a day, you get a clear and realistic picture of the amount of time you available to do the things you need to do. You will see that you need at least 6 hours of sleep. The remaining 18 hours are what remains for other activities. Of these 18 hours, you will go to school most days for about 8 hours a day, which means that you only have approximately 10 hours left for other things. During these 10 hours, you need to account for the time it takes to get ready, transport yourself to different places, eat, and shower. Let's say that together these things take 4 hours. The total time left, in our example, is 6 hours—this is the time you have remaining for your studies. Even if you spend 12 hours in school, you still have 2 hours left to study each day. And if you use these 2 hours well, you can accomplish a lot. As you can see, 6 hours of study time is quite a lot if you use the time well. How is it, then, that we often complain that we don't have enough time? The answer is poor planning and time management[1,2].

In fact, every day you are already unconsciously planning how to use your time. You know when to arrive at school, when to go home to study, and when to get into bed. You also often know when your classes and rotations start. So you are already doing some rough planning in your head. However, from now on, your planning must be a lot more detailed and *written down* because you need to be able to perform well in a short period of time. You don't want to leave anything up to chance.

Planning Your Day

Now you know that planning your day is key. You also know that you need to manage your time well each day. Moreover, you know that on most of the days, you will have at least a few hours of study time. In order to succeed in medical school, get the best grades and scores, and perform well on your rotations, you must plan what, when, and how much you should do during each course and rotation every single day[1-3]. Below, I will teach you some structured planning rules that worked extremely well for me and many other successful medical students[2,3]:

- What should you do and how much time do you have to do it?
- How much time should you spend on each task?
- How much time do *you* need?
- What is most important?

STEP 1. WHAT SHOULD YOU DO AND HOW MUCH TIME DO YOU HAVE TO DO IT?

The first step is to figure out *what* you have to do. If you're starting a new course, find out what all the course material is and what the evaluation criteria are (assignments, quizzes, exams, etc.). Then find out how much time you have to finish each task. If you're starting a new rotation, find out what your schedule is: When do you start in the morning? When do you finish? Do you have any presentations? Breaks? Assignments? See the example in Box 6.1.

STEP 2. HOW MUCH TIME SHOULD YOU SPEND ON EACH TASK?

Step two in your planning involves finding out exactly what you need to do for each task: the number of pages you should read before a quiz or an exam; the number of problems you need to solve before a test; or the amount of information you need to collect in order to write a paper or do a presentation. The point is that you need to sit down and research exactly how much you need to do for the task at hand. Once you know what you need to do and exactly how much time each task will take, you can plan how much time you should devote each day to each task. See the example in Box 6.2.

> **BOX 6.1 ■ Example of Step 1. What Should You Do and How Much Time Do You Have to Do It?**
>
> You are starting your first course in anatomy. The teacher mentions that during this course you will have three quizzes and a final exam at the end. She gives you an information sheet where the dates for the different quizzes and the final exam are stated. The information sheet also states which chapters in the book will be covered by each quiz. This information is key to your planning. You now have clear understanding of what you need to do (which chapters you need to read and study for each quiz and exam) and how much time you have to finish them (the date for each test).
>
> Next, start writing down the deadlines for when you have to finish reading the chapters. Only now can you see how much time you have between each deadline, giving you a rough idea of how much you should do before each quiz. For instance, will you have three chapters to finish before the first quiz in 3 months or do you have 1 month to finish five chapters? You will realize that the latter requires much more time from you. In conclusion, you should always start off by finding out *exactly* what you have to do and when you have to do it.

> **BOX 6.2 ■ Example of Step 2. How Much Time Should You Spend on Each Task?**
>
> You have a quiz on the physiology of the heart. This quiz covers four chapters in your physiology book, and the quiz is in 8 weeks. Each chapter is about 20 pages. That means you have $4 \times 20 = 80$ pages to read, comprehend, and remember before the quiz 8 weeks away. Note that when the quiz is more than 3 weeks away, I recommend that you count for 1 week less than the actual deadline just so you can have a *safety net* in case you need to do some last-minute preparations. In this example, you should account for 7 weeks to grasp the knowledge contained in these 80 pages:
>
> Number of days available to study: 7 weeks × 7 days/week = 49 days
> Number of pages to read per day: 80 pages/49 days = 1.6 pages/day
>
> However, you will likely need to read the 80 pages more than once, so let us jump to step 3.

STEP 3. HOW MUCH TIME DO YOU NEED?

How long does it take *you* to prepare for each task or to learn more than 90% of the content? Some need to read a text twice, while others have to read the same content 10 times in order to remember and understand it. Some need more time to learn pharmacology than anatomy. And some may need to solve problems in the book multiple times, while others need to solve it only once in order to fully understand grasp how to do it. Therefore, this step requires you to reflect honestly on your own abilities so that you can identify how much it takes *you* to comprehend and remember the content. Only *you* know your own abilities—so figure out how much time *you* need to complete each task by the deadline. See the example in Box 6.3.

> **BOX 6.3 ■ Example of Step 3. How Much Time Do *You* Need?**
>
> You have an exam in medical genetics in 4 weeks. The content you'll be tested on includes 30 pages from the book. You know that *you* have to read through all the pages at least three times to remember and understand the text. This means that you have to be able to read a total of 90 pages in 3 weeks (remember to save the last week for last-minute preparation). So, you will need to read 30 pages per week, which means reading about 4 to 5 pages per day (30 pages/7 days) to be able to review the material three times.

STEP 4. PRIORITIZE—WHAT IS MOST IMPORTANT?

In medical school, you will typically have more than just one or two courses to tackle at the same time. You will also have several different assignments, exams, and quizzes within different courses at the same time each semester. This means that you may constantly have multiple deadlines to account for in your planning. Therefore, you must learn to assess which of these tasks and deadlines are most important to address first and thus prioritize. Prioritizing your deadlines is another key factor in the planning process. To prioritize your tasks effectively, you have to consider all the planning rules I just described and then decide what is most important to do first.

Don't spend more time on a task than you need to. Instead, you should spend more time on tasks that are more challenging and difficult for you and less time on topics you know you comprehend easily. Make sure you spend more time on areas where you are weaker. Always plan your work so that the things you have to spend more time on are prioritized first, while the tasks you feel that you can handle more easily are lower on your list of priorities. One exception here: you should always prioritize the *earlier* deadlines. See the example in Box 6.4.

Following Your Plan

A plan is made to be followed. There is no point in creating a plan if you're not going to follow it religiously. Sometimes we will fall behind, but it is essential that you keep up with your plan from day one. In order to maintain the pace and rhythm of your plan, you need to make an accurate plan, and make it as soon as possible. Do not wait to make your plan a few days before a deadline—it is often too late by then. Another tip is to plan in such a way that your preparations

---

BOX 6.4 ■ Example of STEP 4. Prioritize—What is Most Important?

In 4 weeks, you have exams in histology, immunology, and pathology as well as two submissions in microbiology and biochemistry. To review the previous steps:
- Step 1: Start by finding out what the content of each task is.
- Step 2: Find out when each deadline is.
- Step 3: Organize the content and estimate when and what you need to do each day during the limited time you have.
- Step 4. Assess how much time *you* need for repetition or to complete the submissions.

To prioritize, you need to:
- Write down each deadline and task.
  - Exam: Histology; 48 chapters. Deadline: 2 weeks.
  - Exam: Immunology; 40 pages. Deadline: 3 weeks.
  - Exam: Pathology; 55 pages. Deadline: 4 weeks.
  - Submission: Microbiology; write about gram-positive bacteria. Deadline: 2 weeks.
  - Submission: Biochemistry; write about DNA replication. Deadline: 4 weeks.
- For tasks like paper submissions, essays, or presentations, assess how much work you need to do for each of them by doing a thorough analysis of, for instance, what information you need to collect to write up your work.
- Then estimate how much time *you* need to spend on each task to meet each deadline.
- Now think about how to prioritize your deadlines. If you really enjoy histology but dislike pathology or find immunology very difficult, you should spend more time on the latter two and also prioritize them first in your planning. But watch out! Your deadlines for your histology exam and microbiology submission are sooner than the other deadlines. This means that you need to prioritize these as well. Thus, when you prioritize your studies, you need to think about two things: (1) which deadlines come first and (2) which deadlines are more pressing based on your strengths, weaknesses, and workload.

are done a few days to a week before a deadline. As explained earlier, by being well prepared, you are giving yourself a margin of up to a week to do a last-minute review if needed[4].

Write Down Your Plan

Your plan should be in writing. Never try to make a plan in your head! There is no chance that you can keep track of all the chapters, topics, pages, tasks, assignments, information, and deadlines in your head. And even if you could, it is an unnecessary burden on your brain. You should write down your plan on a piece of paper or in your calendar in an organized way so that it's easy to follow. It should be as detailed and accurate as possible, preferably including the exact times when you will start and finish each task. By doing so, you will save yourself time by always knowing exactly *what* to do and *when* to do it.

Keep a copy of your plan on your desk, on your bedroom door, in your phone, and wherever else you spend a lot of time. That way, your plan is always visible and you are constantly reminded of what to do and when to do it. Once you see your plan in front of you, it also means that you can easily follow and stick to it[3,4].

A Plan is Changeable

Remember that a plan is changeable and needs to be adapted as time goes on. There will be new tasks that will come your way, and you need to fit them into your plan and prioritize them. Therefore, it is extremely important that you review your plan regularly, even daily, to evaluate it. A plan is not fixed the way a schedule in school is. Your plan is there for you to keep track of all the important things you need to do now and in the future. It therefore needs to be updated to match your present circumstances. If you receive unplanned assignments in the middle of the week, you should always consider adjusting your plan if need be. All new deadlines that emerge over time should be included, and therefore your plan will be constantly adjusted.

Five Minutes is a Lot of Time

What do you usually do when you have 5 minutes of downtime? Most people use it to rest and do lazy things. Certainly, it is important to recover and take breaks, but there are many times when we have 5 minutes and don't use it productively. Wasting six 5-minutes breaks each day means that you will have wasted 30 minutes in a week. That is 900 minutes, or 15 hours, each month. You might waste even more than that. My mentor once said that if I read every time that I had a break, even for a couple of minutes, I would get a lot more reading done. So I started using every short break to read and, lo and behold, I discovered that my mentor was right.

Try it for yourself: each time you have 5 minutes of downtime, do something productive. Pick up your textbook and start reading, continue to work on your assignments, or do something else of value. How you spend your periodic 5-minute breaks will be a determining factor in what you will achieve in school and in life. Every little bit counts[5].

When You Fall Behind in Your Plan

You will likely encounter days that do not go according to schedule. It's normal and unavoidable. The most common issues that can cause you to veer off course are described below. Make sure to address these issues as soon as possible when you fall behind in your plan[6,7].

YOU PUT TOO MUCH INTO YOUR PLAN

Review your plan again to see whether you assigned yourself too much work at once. See if you can reorganize some of the assignments or tasks that are less urgent. Perhaps you wrote down a task too early in your plan and that can be moved to the following week? Or perhaps you need fewer rounds of repetition on a particular subject? Any chance you can add some downtime to your schedule? Consider the options and revise your plan accordingly.

YOU HAVE LESS TIME THAN YOU THOUGHT

You misjudged the amount of time you have at your disposal. This is a common mistake. Review your overall plan, individual tasks, and deadlines and adjust your schedule to avoid missing a deadline or running out of study time.

YOU STARTED TOO LATE

If your plan says you should start studying on Monday at 4:00 pm, then that's what you should do. Otherwise, you will fall behind because you likely already have something else planned for Tuesday. If you don't start studying until Tuesday, then you have a whole day's worth of work to catch up on. Unfinished tasks can add up very quickly, so my advice is to always start early and never start too late. If you are always starting too late, then consider adjusting your plan. Maybe you need an earlier bedtime or a power nap to reenergize yourself? Look at what might be missing from your plan. You should be able to finish you daily to-do list every day before going to bed.

YOU CREATED YOUR PLAN TOO LATE

As I stated earlier, make sure you create your plan right from the start. Don't wait to do this because work accumulates very quickly and can easily get out of hand. Do your future self a favor and create your plan as soon as possible.

YOU HAVE AN EMERGENCY

Unforeseen events will arise. It can be unexpected visits to the doctor or dentist or family issues. Life goes on while you are in medical school, and you can never be sure what tomorrow will bring. This is another common reason why students fall behind. Therefore, if and when an emergency occurs and you cannot follow your plan, then make sure you catch up as soon as possible. Another tip is to start earlier than the plan states. Last of all, if you finish your to-do list one day early, then start with the next day's tasks so you have some wiggle room to deal with the unexpected.

Summary

- Time is finite and the key limiting resource in medical school. We usually think that we have more time than we do, so make sure that you use your time well.
- You must have an accurate plan during your medical school years. It keeps you on track and increases your likelihood of success.
- To create a plan, follow these four steps:
  - What should you do and how much time do you have to do it?
  - How much time should you spend on each task?
  - How much time do you need?
  - Prioritize—What is most important?

- Create and follow your plan from day one.
- Your plan should be written down on a piece of paper or in a calendar and posted in visible locations.
- Make a realistic plan and follow it. If you fall behind, make sure to catch up as soon as possible.
- A plan can and should constantly be adjusted to remain accurate and useful to you.
- Five minutes is a lot of time—take advantage of every small break in a valuable way.

References

1. Jackson VP. Time management: a realistic approach. *J Am Coll Radiol.* 2009;6(6):434–436. https://doi.org/10.1016/j.jacr.2008.11.018.
2. Schrager S, Sadowski E. Getting more done: strategies to increase scholarly productivity. *J Grad Med Educ.* 2016;8(1):10–13. https://doi.org/10.4300/JGME-D-15-00165.1.
3. Gordon CE, Borkan SC. Recapturing time: a practical approach to time management for physicians. *Postgrad Med J.* 2014;90(1063):267–272. https://doi.org/10.1136/postgradmedj-2013-132012.
4. Brunicardi FC, Hobson FL. Time management: a review for physicians. *J Natl Med Assoc.* 1996;88(9):581–587.
5. Kressin NR, Saha S, Weaver F, Rubenstein L, Weinberger M. Career and time management strategies for clinical and health services researchers. *J Gen Intern Med.* 2007;22(10):1475–1478. https://doi.org/10.1007/s11606-007-0337-7.
6. Gedzelman CF. Falling Behind in School? Some Tips to Catch Up and Become More Organized. Tutoring for Success. http://tutoringforsuccess.us/falling-behind-in-school-some-tips-to-catch-up-and-become-more-organized/. Accessed September 17, 2020.
7. Lucier KL. What to Do When You're Behind in Your College Classes. ThoughtCo.com. https://www.thoughtco.com/what-to-do-if-you-are-behind-in-classes-793164. Published December 7, 2019.

CHAPTER 7

Accelerated Learning

Education is the passport to the future, for tomorrow belongs to those who prepare for it today.

—Malcolm X

What is Accelerated Learning?

Accelerated learning (AL) is an intensive method consisting of study techniques that enable information to be learned in a relatively short time. It was first described at Stanford University in 1986 but has since been evolved to include many different learning techniques that improve understanding, learning, and retention of knowledge[1].

The purpose of AL is to involve as much of the brain as possible and to engage the student in the learning process. Thus, both the right and left sides of the brain are engaged as well as the limbic system and the cortex (lower and higher brain). Studies on AL have shown that when you engage different parts of the brain, information retention and comprehension becomes easier, more natural, and more powerful[1].

The Science Behind Accelerated Learning

There are many different study techniques out there, some better than others. In fact, some of these techniques are low yield, yet they are still frequently used by many students. Therefore, it is critical to understand which methods have been scientifically proven to work and which work best for the majority of students so that you can incorporate the right ones into your studying.

The basis of AL is that knowledge is *created* in the mind rather than merely absorbed. The creation of new patterns, information, meanings, and neural networks happens when you integrate new knowledge into your existing baseline structure or self. Studies also show that optimal learning happens when instruction is more activity based rather than presentation based[2].

AL techniques engage students on many levels simultaneously, taking advantage of all the body's senses. Since the brain works like a parallel processor, not a sequential one, it functions best when it is fully engaged with doing many things at once during the learning process. Consequently, optimal learning occurs when your brain is absorbing many things at once rather than one thing at a time in a linear fashion[2].

There are many benefits to AL but the main ones are as follows[3]:

- You will learn more in less time
- Less effort is required in the learning process
- The learning process is said to be more enjoyable, and
- Learning this way is more productive.

Accelerated Learning Techniques for Faster Comprehension and Retention

While AL is used at many institutions and studies show that it can be effective, AL might not work for everyone. Since this book is meant to be a comprehensive guide to helping you succeed in your studies, I will describe some of the AL techniques that are in use today so you can try them out for yourself. You can even try combining different techniques from the different sections of this book. Once you know what the most frequently used methods are, you can test which ones work best for you in each of your courses[4-7].

SET GOALS

AL starts with the basic principle of setting goals and objectives for what you want to learn. As I explained in Chapter 5, goal setting is a major factor in being successful. You have to know where you want to go in order to get there. This is not only true for succeeding in your studies but also other areas of life. Goal setting is often underrated and omitted by many students. Goal setting does not just involve big achievements in life but can include anything that you want to accomplish. Therefore, start each study session by setting appropriate goals and objectives for what you want to accomplish with a chapter, book, course, and so on. Proper goal setting in this situation involves:

- Goals that are realistic to accomplish
- Goals that are clear and well defined
- Goals that you actually want to achieve
- Goals that matter to you and have a clear "why"
- Goals that help you grow, and
- Goals that include the 80/20 rule (see below).

Once you've set your goals, you can divide them into smaller goals like stepping-stones. This process is described in Chapter 5 on goal setting.

BLOCK OUT DISTRACTIONS

AL is all about focusing on one thing at a time. After you've set your goals, it's time to focus on achieving one goal at a time. In order to focus, you need to remove all distractions. Clear your desk and turn off all electronics. That means no YouTube, no social media, no emailing, no texting. You can try doing two things at the same time, but your attention will be divided and the quality of your results will go down. Much of the time, multitasking on goals makes you unproductive.

USE MEMORY TECHNIQUES

I have outlined many different memory and learning techniques in this book. Use them to systematically learn all the new knowledge presented to you in each of your courses. The best way to learn something new is to first learn the system that goes with it. Learn the system well, then practice, practice, practice. For example, when you want to try a new recipe, you first read through the instructions a few times. You might watch a tutorial or two. Only then do you start to prepare the ingredients and cook them in the proper order. If you just started to mix the different ingredients together without having first read and understood the recipe, you might end up with a meal at the end, but it would likely take you much longer to prepare and be far from superior in taste and appearance. Therefore, be sure to learn all the study techniques the right way before you embark on learning something new. Then it's just a matter of practice, practice, practice.

TRY MIND MAPPING

Mind mapping is an old concept. It helps you organize information in a simple visual format. It also helps you to correlate multiple things together by structuring information in categories. The visual element of this AL technique also enhances your learning. Mind maps can help you break down more complex problems into smaller, more digestible parts.

PRACTICE NEW SKILLS

When you learn something new, put it into practice right away. AL involves actively practicing your new knowledge. That way, the information sticks much better in the brain. For instance, if you learn about stroke, try to practice it in a clinical setting; bring it to the bedside, and think about the symptoms, diagnosis, and treatment when you see patients. The same thing goes with every bit of knowledge you learn. Once you learn something new, do your best to put it into practice by using the information rather than just repeating it in your head.

FOLLOW THE 80/20 RULE

The 80/20 rule—also known as the Pareto principle, the law of the vital few, or the principle of factor sparsity—states that about 80% of the effects from many events come from 20% of the causes. This principle is often used in many other fields. For instance, in business it is said that 80% of sales come from 20% of customers. In many languages, 20% of the words make up 80% of the written language. In music, 80% of all pop songs come from 20% of all chord progressions. The same goes with your studies to some degree: 80% of your results will come from 20% of your work[6].

Now, I'm not saying that you should learn only 20% of the course material. But just having this principle in mind may change your perspective on your course material. You see, many times we talk about how certain information in a course is the most important to know. And this is true—there will always be facts in different courses that are must-knows. And yes, you should still learn all the material presented to you and use all the study techniques that work for you. However, you can be sure that, sometimes, knowing the most important things, perhaps the vital 20%, means that you might know 80% of all the most commonly encountered problems in a course.

STUDY WITH FRIENDS

You've likely heard of the saying that two minds are better than one. While this is not always true, it can be useful to study with other students, the ones who have the same mindset and mentality and are at least as ambitious as you. They could teach you certain things you don't know, explain complex ideas, or simply assist you in the learning process. It also helps your mind to better retain information when you discuss topics out loud.

Studying with your classmates enables you to benefit from one another's abilities and acquire skills together. The most important thing, however, is to study with students that are focused, motivated, and take things seriously. This is not a joke or play session. It is a study session. Thus, it is important that you set the objectives of what you will study, how you will study, and for how long you will study before the session begins. It's also important to maintain focus throughout the session. If one of you loses focus, then you can help each other get back on track.

TRACK YOUR PROGRESS

Track your progress by keeping a record of each study session and how long it is. That's the principle behind data analytics, a fancy term that means analyzing data and drawing conclusions from it. In medical school, as in life, if you don't know where you are, you don't know where you're going. The same principle applies to your studies. You have to track how much you've studied and what you've learned. Data analytics is used in sports and business all the time. In fact, in business, there are departments that focus only on data analytics. What gets measured gets managed. This is one of the fundamental principles of AL. To track your progress, you need to:

- Write down exactly everything you have studied in a session
- Write down the things you have learned from the study session, and
- Align this information with your plan to make sure you are on track.

TAKE BREAKS

Medical school is often overwhelming and difficult. Your days will be filled with long lectures, practice sessions, rotations, and self-studying. This could easily lead to burnout. Therefore, it is essential that you take breaks in between your study sessions. It is not only about burnout either—studying too long without breaks also affects your productivity, memory, and learning. However, taking a break for just 5 to 10 minutes each hour can refresh your mind and reenergize you. Most people work most efficiently in 25- to 60-minute sessions rather than 4 to 5 hours straight. However, regardless of how long you are able to work, please be sure to take breaks. Reasonable breaks are not a waste of time, as they can actually help you study longer and retain information better. During the breaks, you can do anything from just sitting and doing nothing to taking a power nap, meditating, or eating a healthy snack. Whatever you do, it should be the total opposite of studying so your mind can relax for a little while.

Summary

- Accelerated learning (AL) is an intensive method consisting of study techniques that enable information to be learned in a relatively short time.
- Studies have shown that AL can improve your learning and actually make you learn faster and more efficiently.
- AL is not for everyone; however, you should know what it is, try it out, and see whether it works for you. If it does work, then use AL or incorporate it with other study methods.

References

1. Hopfenberg WS, Levin HM. *Accelerated Schools.* School of Education: Stanford University; 1990.
2. Meier D. *The Accelerated Learning Handbook: A Creative Guide to Designing and Delivering Faster, More Effective Training Programs.* McGraw-Hill Education; 2000.

3. Accelerated Learning. The Peak Performance Center. http://thepeakperformancecenter.com/educational-learning/learning/theories/accelerated-learning/. Accessed September 16, 2020.

4. Bunkley N. Joseph Juran, 103, pioneer in quality control, dies. *New York Times.* March 3, 2008. Accessed 25 January 2018. https://www.nytimes.com/2008/03/03/business/03juran.html.

5. Box GEP, Meyer RD. An analysis for unreplicated fractional factorials. *Technometrics.* 1986;28(1):11–18. https://doi.org/10.2307/1269599.

6. Marshall P. The 80/20 Rule of Sales: How to Find Your Best Customers. Entrepreneur.com. https://www.entrepreneur.com/article/229294. Published October 9, 2013. Accessed May 1, 2018.

7. Jarrett N. 5 Useful Accelerated Learning Techniques. edtech4beginners.com. https://edtech4beginners.com/2017/04/13/guest-post-5-useful-accelerated-learning-techniques/. Published April 13, 2017.

CHAPTER 8

Lecture Time in Medical School

When people talk, listen completely. Most people never listen.
Ernest Hemingway

Most of the successful people I've known are the ones who do more listening than talking.
Bernard M. Baruch

Why Class Time is Different in Medical School

By now you should understand some of the ways in which medical school is different from other programs. Indeed, all university programs have their own unique features. A defining feature of health care programs like medicine is their emphasis on ensuring students' deep understanding of a wide range of topics. In many other programs, you can more easily get away with learning surface-level information or memorizing formulas to solve financial or economic problems. In medicine, however, there is no one-size-fits-all approach to the patients you will see and their health issues. Patients have unique genetics and biology, so the presentation of their symptoms can often be atypical. Therefore, in order to become a good physician, you must first comprehend—at a level of understanding that far exceeds memorization—how different mechanisms in the body interact with each other. Once you do, you will become more confident in using your knowledge in the management of patients.

Many topics in medical school are incredibly complex. It takes time to fully comprehend each course on different aspects of the human body, whereas learning a formula and plugging in numbers doesn't involve the same level of difficulty. This doesn't mean that other programs are not challenging; it simply means that in medicine there is a different approach to learning information and applying it. Even with the dozens of new sophisticated medical apps and online resources designed to guide physicians in making accurate diagnoses and choosing appropriate treatments, *the physician* is still the one responsible for being discerning and making good decisions. Given the responsibility you will one day bear for your patients' health, you should take the greatest care to ensure that your learning in medical school is optimal.

The Value of Lecture Time for Health Care Courses

Class or lecture time in medical school has many benefits. Most information that you need to know about a topic is presented to you in class by your professors. They will also emphasize what is most important to learn, allowing you to make the best use of your time outside of class. Since your professors are delivering the information that you will eventually be tested on, ensure that you are paying attention and absorbing all the knowledge with 100% focus.

Imagine you're at an expensive restaurant: You order a meal and pay for it, then leave the food at the restaurant and go home to cook a meal for yourself—probably something not even half as good. You would never do that! The same principle applies to classes in medical school. If you don't go to class, or if you do attend class but don't stay focused, you will have to go home and acquire all the knowledge on your own. So take advantage of classes. If you do not, you might as well start cooking your own food after paying for your uneaten restaurant meals as well, which I think you'll agree is absurd[1].

The Art of Listening

Without a doubt, effective listening will save you time, effort, and likely improve your results and academic skills. Picture yourself sitting in a class for 2 hours where all the information is presented to you. You have two choices: you can actively listen and attempt to grasp the information or you can let you mind drift to other things. The latter approach will force you to gather all the information by yourself later on, which means that you have just wasted 2 hours of your time. The former approach, however, gives you the first round of learning.

But what is learning, and how does information stick in your mind? We learn through repetition. Some people may have to read a text 10 times, others only twice. Regardless of how many times you have to repeat something in order for the information to stick, the learning process always begins with the first time you hear or see information. And it is always better to first *hear* information and *then* start reading about it, because you get to hear a topic actually explained to you[2,3].

Therefore, in class, you should actively listen to the teacher. This is not easy. Listening is an active process that takes energy from you. Have you ever wondered why browsing through Instagram or Facebook is so easy and satisfying? It's partly because it does not consume much energy. As you passively scroll down a screen to see new status updates or images, you do not need to interpret the information or make meaning of it. However, listening to someone speak requires that you focus on hearing their words, taking in the information, understanding it, and then return to listening to the next thing they are saying. Of course this cognitive activity demands more energy than scrolling through Instagram.

Think about how much you listen to someone whenever you are in class: 20% of the time? 50%? Or perhaps even less? You will discover that listening attentively is hard work. Maybe you haven't yet understood why listening is so important, so you haven't paid attention in the past. Maybe you have not yet developed this skill. Either way, listening is a skill that anyone can practice and master[2,3]. Here are a few tips on how to be a good listener[4]:

1. **The most important person in your life.** Imagine yourself meeting the most important person in the world to you. You are lucky enough to have a 1-hour conversation with them. Who would you choose? Whoever it is, I assure you that you will be hanging onto every word they say. You will have your ears perked and will be giving that person your undivided attention. Now think about the classroom: Do you think you show the same attentiveness to your teachers? Most of us don't. From now on, to make the most out of your education, you need to treat your teachers as the most important people in your life. Once you do, you will automatically start listening better. In turn, better listening will lead you to remember and learn things better and therefore get better results.

2. **Maintain eye contact and face the teacher.** It is much easier to listen when you are facing someone and making eye contact with them. By keeping your body position in mind, you will be less likely to think about unrelated things or look at and get distracted by your phone. Being distracted by other things is one of the major reasons why we don't listen attentively. As soon as you get distracted, intentionally refocus your mind by looking at your teacher.

3. **Remove all distractions.** We often do not listen well because we allow ourselves to get distracted. That distraction could be your phone, your wandering thoughts, or your books and your papers in front of you. Whatever it is, remember to put those items away, out of sight. Make sure that your classroom time becomes an active listening session where nothing can distract you. Put your phone on silent and all your other books and papers—all you need in class is your notebook, your pen, and your focus.

4. **Be present.** Being present is difficult for many students. This means that you should not react to your thoughts the way you typically do. During a lecture, there will be many thoughts, feelings, and sensations running through you. This is natural, but we do not have to react to or focus on them. Instead, whenever you feel like you are getting caught up in a thought, feeling, or sensation, just notice it, then let it go and refocus your attention back on the teacher, back to what is happening in the present. Regardless of how you are feeling that day—happy, sad, angry, or something else—the key is not to get rid of the feelings or thoughts. Instead, train yourself not to react. You cannot help how you feel or think, but you *can* choose how you to respond. The more your practice this technique, the better you will be at being present and listening.

5. **Be attentive—pay attention.** Pay attention to what the teacher is saying, how that is related to what you are learning, how you are going to grasp this information, and how the information is being given to you. Try to filter out all distractions, like the person next to you and background noise or activity. Don't pay attention to anything else except the person who is talking in front of you—your teacher.

6. **Listen with an open mind.** Do not judge or jump to conclusions about what and how the teacher is saying something. That will just distract you. Instead, focus on taking in the information and writing good notes. Remember that the teacher is usually the expert in the area, so you do not need to reach any conclusions at that point. If you have questions, feel free to ask. But ask questions to make yourself understand something better, not to prove the other person wrong.

7. **Listen using images.** To augment your learning, try to come up with funny mental pictures to accompany the lecture topic. Allow your mind to create a memorable image. You are more likely to remember and understand information that way.

The Art of Focusing

People have different attention spans. Depending on how long yours is, you will find yourself getting tired after a certain amount of focusing[5]. People's attention spans last anywhere from a few minutes to an hour, but thereafter we all need a break. However, it is possible to train your attention span to get better. Improving it is crucial in order to be able to listen closely during lectures and also to retain information. The first step is to become aware of the need to improve your focusing skills and make a conscious decision to invest the time and energy needed to improve it.[5]

Many students don't consider focus a strategic skill, so they do not bother examining how good their focus is. When you don't treat it as a strategic issue, deprioritizing its importance is easy, and soon you may ignore it completely.[5] Below are tips on how you can improve your focus:

1. **Reflect on your focus.** Make an inventory of how well you focus during the day. Is your focus time optimal for 5 minutes or an hour? Do you get distracted easily? How many minutes do you lose per day because of distractions? These are questions you need to ask yourself and answer honestly. You need an accurate baseline so that you know what to aim for. Thus, reflect and make notes on your baseline focus. Log your activities for a week. Write down your to-do list each day and log each distraction you experience and the time you spend on distractions. This will give you a clear picture of how often and for how long you get distracted[5].

2. **Avoid distractions.** This is stating the obvious. You need to avoid distractions during your years in medical school. This is something you need to train yourself to do, because our smartphones, constant notifications, and the 24-hour news cycle make it easy to get and stay distracted all day long. Your ability to focus is thought to be directly proportional to how well you can avoid distractions. You become distracted when you allow thoughts to enter your mind that remove your attention from the important task in hand. It is natural to get distracted; I get distracted too. However, the important thing is to limit the distractions you have control over. It is also critical to recognize how *much* you actually do get distracted and train your mind to get less distracted. It's about establishing priorities. To do that effectively, you have to be able to control the external distractions that will inevitably bombard you[5].

3. **Meditate.** Studies show that meditation is one of the best ways to improve your focus and concentration. Meditation is mental training for your attention. Just like you train your muscles in the gym, meditation trains your "brain muscles" and improves your attention span. With meditation, you are essentially training your "monkey" mind not to get distracted by, or react to, the stream of thoughts that are generated by your mind itself. One study showed that students who meditated for 10 to 20 minutes a day, four times a week, for 2 weeks, had higher scores on memory tests[6,7].

4. **Exercise.** Exercise is good for your overall health. But it has also been shown to improve your focus. One study showed that students with attention-deficit/hyperactivity disorder (ADHD) who performed moderate exercise for 20 minutes daily were able to score better on tests and pay more attention[8].

5. **Drink water.** Being dehydrated is not just bad for your health, but also affects your focus. Even mild dehydration can negatively impact your focus. Make sure that you always have a full water bottle by your side and that you sip water throughout the day[9].

6. **Take careful notes.** Taking good notes during lecture gives you the opportunity to not get distracted and also allows for more complete recall later. And when I say take notes, I am talking about doing your best to quote your teacher. The more accurately you record what your teacher says, the more focused you will be, and the less likely it is that you will miss anything. After lecture, you can re-read the majority of what your teacher said. Some also suggest taking notes by hand instead of using a laptop, since your computer may distract you in other ways—texting, social media, emails, and so on. Whatever method you choose, make sure you are just taking notes and nothing else. This will keep you focused.

7. **Chew gum.** Some studies show that chewing gum increases our attention span. This may or may not work for you, but it's worth a try. I know for a fact that it *does* work for me. Whatever you do, chew quietly[10].

8. **Set a focus goal.** You can't run a marathon the first day you start running. Likewise, you cannot expect that your focus will be perfect the first few times you try. It takes practice. The first few times, you may only be able to focus for a few minutes. But the more you practice focusing, the better you will get. So start by setting a goal of focusing for 10 minutes. And then increase it by 5 minutes at a time until you reach your "sweet spot" of concentration, somewhere between 25 and 60 minutes.

9. Whenever you have a break, make sure you stand up, stretch, and restore the blood circulation. You should probably not do this if you are in a lecture and your teacher is talking, but as soon as you get a break, stretching and moving around a bit helps with blood circulation and can improve your focus.

The Art of Note-Taking

During lecture, your teacher usually writes down and talks about the most important things you should know. Everything that is written down or talked about is often high-yield and something you should take notes on in a structured way to read about later on.

Writing good notes is an art. Not everyone can do it well. But if you learn how to do it well, you will benefit immensely. I know a handful of students that relied on studying only their own notes and successfully passed their exams[11,12].

Taking notes allows you to solve two major challenges during lecture. The first challenge is that your memory and what you can reliably retain from a lecture is rather limited. Therefore, your notes allow you to review and recall information later on. The second challenge is what we discussed earlier: limitations in your ability to focus. Taking notes lets you focus on the lecture, which can last several hours. There will be days where you are tired and sleepy, and just relaxing during lecture may be tempting. However, you cannot get lazy or let your sleepiness affect your learning. Take notes so that you remain active and alert despite your tiredness[11,12].

Taking notes, especially good ones, is not easy. We have to listen to our teacher's words, focus on what they are saying, make a conclusion, and then write it down. This can be overwhelming if you have not yet learned how to take good notes. There are many different note-taking techniques, and you need to experiment to find the one that fits you best. Here are a few different note-taking methods for you to try, along with their pros and cons[13]:

CORNELL METHOD

This method systematically divides notes into four parts: (1) main notes, (2) main ideas and keywords, (3) questions, and (4) summary. In the main notes section, you will write down all the notes that you feel are important. In the main ideas and keywords section, you will write down all the important keywords your teacher mentioned. In the questions section, you will write down questions that relate to the notes you've taken. Writing down questions helps to clarify things, reveal relationships, establish continuity, and improve your memory. The writing of questions also sets the stage for studying for exams later. Lastly, you will write down a summary of each section of your notes. This summary is a chance to reflect on and restate the ideas in your own words, which will enhance your learning.

- Pros:
  - Organized way of writing your notes
  - Allows you to reflect on your notes right on the spot
  - Fast way to write, organize, and review your notes
  - Assists you with extracting main ideas
  - Cuts down on review time

- Cons:
  - At times, you may find it hard to identify the keywords.
  - You may not have enough time to reflect, as your teacher will keep talking while you write your summary.
  - You need to prepare your pages in advance of the lecture.

CHARTING METHOD

This method involves organizing information into several columns, where each column represents a category that makes the rows comparable. This method is best to use when there is a lot of information to memorize.

- Pros:
  - Information is structured, organized, and easy to review.
  - Easy to compare, read, and memorize information
- Cons:
  - Time-consuming
  - Difficult to do during lectures where the information is not clear in advance
  - Only works when the information can be categorized

OUTLINE METHOD

This is one of the most common note-taking techniques. It involves writing down notes in point form to cover different topics and subtopics.

- Pros:
  - Excellent method when a lot of information is being presented
  - Allows you to focus more on what your teacher is saying rather than get distracted by the need to structure your notes
  - Clean structure
  - Highlights the main points of the lecture in an organized fashion
- Cons:
  - Not optimal for courses such as biochemistry, where many charts and formulas are involved
  - Difficult to do when the lecture is unstructured

MAPPING METHOD

This method allows you to organize your notes into branches and establish interrelated connections between them. It involves writing down the main topic at the top of the page and subdividing it into subtopics on the right and left as you move down the page.

- Pros:
  - Good for heavy content, where information needs to be organized
  - Enables notes to be visualized, which can help with the learning process
- Cons:
  - You can easily run out of space.
  - May not allow you to cover all the information needed
  - Can be time-consuming to create adequate branches and images

QUOTING METHOD

This method involves trying to write down everything your teacher says verbatim. You will most likely not get every single word, but that is your goal. While some might not like this method, it's the one that I used during medical school. I was able to compile all the information while minimizing the risk of missing anything. It also allowed me to focus better during lecture.

- Pros:
    - Captures most of the content presented to you
    - Helps you maintain optimal focus on what the teacher is saying
    - Good for lectures where most of the content is extremely high-yield
    - Notes become your secondary memory.
- Cons:
    - Takes time and effort
    - Might capture a lot of "unnecessary" information that needs to be filtered out later

SUMMARY OF NOTE-TAKING METHODS

There is no "right" way to take notes. Each of our brains works a little differently when it comes to learning new things, so the right note-taking method for you will come down to preference based on how your brain works. Therefore, I encourage you to try all of the note-taking methods (Table 8.1). When you do, make sure to note which method (1) allows you to feel comfortable taking notes for a long period, (2) gives you enough time to cover most of what the teacher says, and (3) promotes the most effective learning of the content.

The other point to consider is that good note-taking requires practice. No method will come naturally the first few times, so practice note-taking outside lecture time. A simple exercise is to summarize the news. Start by listening to a TV or radio news segment each day and trying each of the different methods to see which one suits you best. Once you settle on a particular method, practice it several times until it becomes second nature.

TABLE 8.1 ■ **Comparison of Different Note-Taking Methods**

Method	Pros	Cons	Website
Cornell method	• Organized way of writing your notes • Allows you to reflect on your notes right on the spot • Fast way to write, organize, and review your notes • Assists you with extracting main ideas • Cuts down on review time	• At times, you may find it hard to identify the keywords. • You may not have enough time to reflect, as your teacher will keep talking while you write your summary. • You need to prepare your pages in advance of the lecture.	http://lsc.cornell.edu/notes.html
Charting method	• Information is structured, organized, and easy to review. • Easy to compare, read, and memorize information	• Time-consuming • Difficult to do during lectures where the information is not clear in advance • Only works when the information can be categorized.	https://www.oxfordlearning.com/5-effective-note-taking-methods/ https://medium.goodnotes.com/the-best-note-taking-methods-for-college-students-451f412e264e

TABLE 8.1 ■ Comparison of Different Note-Taking Methods—cont'd

Method	Pros	Cons	Website
Outline method	• Excellent method when a lot of information is being presented • Allows you to focus more on what your teacher is saying rather than get distracted by the need to structure your notes • Clean structure • Highlights the main points of the lecture in an organized fashion	• Not optimal for courses such as biochemistry, where many charts and formulas are involved • Difficult to do when the lecture is unstructured	https://www.missouristate.edu/assets/busadv/p.24.pdf https://medium.goodnotes.com/the-best-note-taking-methods-for-college-students-451f412e264e
Mapping method	• Good for heavy content, where information needs to be organized • Enables notes to be visualized, which can help with the learning process	• You can easily run out of space. • May not allow you to cover all the information needed • Can be time-consuming to create adequate branches and images	https://www.ncbi.nlm.nih.gov/pmc/articles/PMC5348998/
Quoting method	• Captures most of the content presented to you • Helps you maintain optimal focus on what the teacher is saying • Good for lectures where most of the content is extremely high yield • Notes become your secondary memory.	• Takes time and effort • Might capture a lot of "unnecessary" information that needs to be filtered out later	https://www.ncbi.nlm.nih.gov/pmc/articles/PMC4812780/

The Art of Asking Questions

You will occasionally find yourself sitting in lectures where you feel confused or do not understand the content. This is normal. In these situations, your best bet is to ask questions for clarity. It's especially important in the beginning of the lecture, since if you do not understand what has been said in the beginning, you may not understand things later on either. Therefore, I encourage you to ask questions, even if you have many. As the saying goes, there are no stupid questions, only stupid answers. It is important to ask the teacher your many questions. I did that in medical school, and many smart students I know do so as well. Don't be embarrassed by asking a lot, and do not think that people think you are less smart by asking questions. A lot of students are inhibited by their fear of being judged for asking many questions. But in reality, no one cares that much and in fact, when people do ask questions, it shows a level of involvement, interest, and intelligence. Chances are that other people in the class have the same questions, too.

Here are some tips on asking good questions[14,15]:

1. **Prepare questions.** You will likely know what topics will be addressed in future lectures. Briefly looking at the content in your book and reflecting on the topic allows you to

formulate questions. Preparing questions in advance gives you time to reflect on the content and will also make you retain the answer better.

2. **Ask questions you don't know the answers to.** Although there may be times when you ask a question in order to seek confirmation or clarification, the best questions are those that you don't know the answers to and come from genuine curiosity. In case time is limited, those are the most important questions to ask.

3. **Formulate the question well.** If you want a broad answer, then ask an open-ended question. If you want to know about a specific thing, then make your question more specific. Remember that the way you ask a question will give you a certain type of answer, so think about how you ask a question so that the answer will satisfy you.

4. **Types of questions.** There are different types of questions aimed at achieving different goals. Once you know what the different types of questions are, it will be easier to ask questions for a more satisfactory answer (Table 8.2).

There are many ways to ask a question. The type of question you ask depends on what you want to get out of your query. Regardless of what the question is, the key is that your question should allow you to better understand something in order to grasp the topic better, retain the information better, and then make decisions based on the knowledge you have. Consequently, you should ask questions—and many of them—but be sure to ask them in the right way.

TABLE 8.2 ■ Types of Test Questions

Question Type	Description	Examples
Clarifying question	A clarifying question will assist you with understanding the full extent of what the teacher has said. This type of question fills in the gaps and allows the teacher to give you a more well-rounded explanation.	"Why is it like that?" "Why do you say so?"
Funneling question	A funneling question adds depth to a topic. It allows you to reach the core of the problem. To fundamentally understand something, you often have to dig deeper into the topic. At the end of the day, things stick in our memory when we fully understand them.	"How was this analysis done?" "How did they carry out this study to achieve these results?"
Adjoining question	With an adjoining question, you can explore how a given topic is related to other areas, which may not always be brought up during lecture.	"How would this relate to other areas?" "How would this be applied in a clinical setting?"
Elevating question	An elevating question explores the topic out of the box. It allows you to emphasize the bigger picture.	"How would the inflammatory cascade affect the overall health both negatively and positively?" "How do we tie all of this together in a clinical setting?"

The Art of Efficiency

We live in a fast-paced world where time constantly feels limited. Technology is both a gift and a curse: it allows us to facilitate information exchange, yet captures our attention and steals our time. We all know how computers, emails, phones, and social media consume a significant part of our day. These and other ubiquitous technologies often keep us from doing valuable things with our time, things that would give us much greater benefits in the future.

The concept of spending your time with valuable tasks is simple. You have to understand the model of return on investment (ROI) and opportunity cost. I like to combine these two concepts in school because they relate to each other and provide the necessary mental models for you to assess your daily choices and how you spend your time. It forces you to think about which activities in your life provide you with the highest ROI and also to consider the cost of spending time on activities with a low ROI[16].

ROI is a performance measure used to evaluate the efficiency of an investment or to compare the efficiency of different investments to one another. Thus, ROI measures what you are getting back on a specific investment[16]. This investment could be money, time, or other things, but for our purposes here, ROI means the time investment in your daily life. As you know, this is an incredibly important measurement for business but it can also be applied to your years in medical school, as time is one of your biggest assets. For instance, if you invest a weekend going on a trip, your return is potentially the happiness and fun that you receive from it. However, if you instead choose to spend a weekend studying for you pharmacology exam, your return will be the knowledge that you receive from the time spent studying that particular section, which then could result in your getting a better grade in that course and knowing more than others.

The definition of opportunity cost is the loss of potential gain from other alternatives when one alternative is chosen (also discussed in Chapter 2)[17]. The reason why this concept is important is because it makes you realize that if you choose one activity instead of another, you will then gain or lose certain things with that choice. Going back to our example, if you spend a weekend travelling, your opportunity cost is the knowledge you likely would have gained from studying at home that weekend. However, the costs can sometimes be even bigger than that. For example, if your exam took place on the Monday right after that weekend and you were not sufficiently prepared, your grade might have been affected as well. Thus, you see that there is a price we pay for the activities that we choose. This price could be less knowledge, less fun, worse grades, and other consequences we cannot foresee. It is therefore very important to think about opportunity cost every single day when you create your to-do list so that you can make the most of your time. Similarly, for each activity that you choose to do, assess the loss of possible gain from other alternatives[17].

In business, calculating the ROI or measuring the opportunity cost can be difficult at times, especially when there are multiple variables to take account for or when the future of the variables is uncertain[16]. In school and your situation, however, it should be relatively easy to weigh going out with friends versus staying in for the night to study. There are few things that will give you a greater ROI than spending most of your time in college and medical school studying in order to acquire the best knowledge, get the best grades, and become a top student. If you are in college, this investment of your time will result in a higher probability that you will get accepted into medical school (if that is what you want); if you are already in medical school, becoming a top student will most likely allow you to match into the specialty you want. These achievements will translate to your being happy, more confident, better compensated at work, and doing what you love to do. However, if you choose to do things that eat into your time for studying and other school activities, then you will have to pay the price (opportunity cost) of potentially losing these things.

Now that you understand the concepts of ROI and opportunity cost, you know that being efficient during your years in medical school is of the utmost importance. The day is only 24 hours long. By necessity, a part of this time goes to sleep, eating, showering, and personal hygiene. The more you can do during the remaining hours of the day, the better. Efficiency means that you are making the best use of your resources with the least amount of time and effort[18]. If you think about it, the more you can use your time to get the necessary things done, with the least amount of effort, the more time you will have for other things.

Here are some things that you, as a student, can do to improve your efficiency[19,20]:

1. **Organize yourself with a plan.** Whenever you find yourself being inefficient, it's because you haven't decided what to do first, second, third, and so on. When this happens, it is easy to feel overwhelmed and disorganized. You may start putting things off because you aren't sure what to do first. As Benjamin Franklin said, "If you fail to plan, you are planning for failure." Everything starts with a plan, a strategy. Starting each morning by thinking about what you want to do is terribly inefficient. The more structure you have to your day, the easier it is for your brain to process things, the more time you will save, and the more productive you will be. Therefore, always create a plan—in advance—for your studies and other important commitments. Chapter 6 gives you an overview of how to create a study plan. Make sure you have a plan and a to-do list every single day.

2. **Take breaks.** Efficiency and productivity are closely related. To be productive, you need to make time for your basic biological need to rest. Typically, we all need a small break after 60 to 90 minutes of studying. At this mark, you need to think about some sort of pause to recharge your batteries before you start the next cycle. And it doesn't really matter where you are in your plan, page, or problem list: after 90 minutes, you should take a break. Otherwise, the information you are studying won't be as meaningful, teachable, or productive. Go for a walk, take a power nap, eat a healthy snack, listen to music, or meditate. Whatever you do, do something other than studying and looking at your phone. But limit your breaks. A break is a break and should not be more than 10 to 15 minutes.

3. **Minimize distractions.** I have mentioned this before, so it does not require much elaboration. Just remember that distractions are the enemy of productivity and efficiency. Remove all distractions that you can think of and focus on the task at hand. As soon as you catch yourself being distracted, refocus on your task.

4. **Set a timer.** One way to know how well you are using your time is to use a timer. Set the timer for 60 minutes and remember that you should not do anything else except concentrate on your work.

5. **Monitor your daily tasks.** How is that some people can be so much more efficient than others in the same 24-hour period? It's because efficient people are conscious of what they are doing *at all times*. They track how they spend their time. Keep a close eye on yourself and write down, in 15-minute increments, how you are using your limited hours. This diary will give you a snapshot of how much time goes to high-value versus low-value tasks and activities such as watching TV, social media, and other unimportant tasks. Keep track of your daily activities and assess their importance, then remove things that are not adding value or are destroying your productivity[21]. Five minutes on YouTube can easily balloon into an hour.

6. **Do the "worst" thing first.** Most people focus best in the morning. You are typically well rested after a good night's sleep and have high cortisol levels and a "fresh" brain. Therefore, you should do the most important and "unpleasant" task in your to-do list first. That will provide the most energy to undertake this task. Moreover, once this task is finished, you will feel a sense of relief and accomplishment, which will give you more confidence to tackle the rest of your list[22].

7. **Do not procrastinate.** Most things that come up during the course of a day are not that important. Your phone rings, you receive a text message, you get an email: these can all be taken care of later. However, people often prioritize these distractions right when they show up. One of the reasons why is because we get hit of dopamine from every ping, ring, and notification: a phone call, text, or email is easier to deal with. These distractions take your mind away from a much harder and more energy-demanding activity like studying. But each time you allow yourself to attend to such a distraction, your focus and attention increasingly dwindle. The solution is to always think about ROI, opportunity cost, and the bigger picture. As humans, we are wired to consider the needs of the present much more strongly than those of the future. This tendency is referred to as "temporal discounting" in psychology. Remember what will give you the most value in life, the highest ROI for your future, and the opportunity cost of your choice to neglect your priorities. Keeping these things in mind will decrease your risk of procrastination[19,20].

The Art of Preparing for Lectures

By now you know that lectures are valuable because the most important information is delivered to you. However, if the topic is completely new to you, it is difficult to absorb all the content. The amount of information that can be retained during a lecture varies from person to person, but there may be lectures where perhaps only 5% to 10% of the content is absorbed and understood.

Logically, it makes that knowing some of the content in advance would be beneficial not just from the standpoint of understanding but also from a memory standpoint[23]. Imagine a topic in your head that you know very well, such as Apple products. Now imagine getting a lecture about iPhones, MacBooks, and iPads. Since you already have baseline knowledge about these products, your understanding and retention of Apple's new features and upgrades will be much easier to understand and remember. Everything that you already know will be an additional round of repetition, and the new knowledge will just build upon your existing foundation.

Your experience would be similar to someone giving me a lecture about myocardial infarction: I would already know most of the content, so hearing it a second time would serve as a round of repetition and strengthen my memory. On the other hand, if I attended a lecture on the elephants of Southern Africa, I would likely be hearing most of it for the first time and therefore learning everything from scratch. And since our minds can absorb only a limited amount of information at once, I would not only learn less but probably also understand the topic in much less detail.

The same goes for lecture time, college, and medical school. The more knowledge and comprehension you already have about a topic, the better you will absorb and remember new knowledge presented to you. The first time you read something new, there will be new concepts and information that are not always clear or easy to understand. Moreover, you won't remember everything in much detail either. But once you attend class and the professor starts lecturing on the same topic you just read about, you will have a different experience: concepts will start to clear up; information will be repeated; questions that may have arisen during your initial reading might get answered; and you may understand things that previously seemed unclear, since you will be hearing the information a second time and in a slightly different way.

If your time allows, take the trouble of preparing for a topic before the lecture, as your learning will be enhanced[23]. There are different ways to prepare. You can read the chapter. You can read the handouts. You can listen to audiotapes about that topic. Or you can simply read about the subject online (on reliable websites, of course). The key is to familiarize yourself with the content so that it is not brand new to you. Again, the more you know in advance, the better you will absorb the new information presented to you. How much you prepare for each lecture will vary and depend on your current knowledge about the topic, how much time you have, and how advanced the new topic is.

For instance, if you are already behind in your plan, you should obviously prioritize your most important tasks and maybe only skim the chapter. If the topic on the lecture is relatively simple and straightforward in your opinion, then you may not need to prepare at all; that would be a poor use of your limited time. By contrast, if you have time or if the topic is complex, preparing for it by reading the chapter once or twice could be beneficial. Therefore, the strategy is to assess your schedule, plan your future lecture topics continuously, and evaluate whether and how much to prepare for each lecture.

Virtual medical teaching in the setting of the COVID-19 pandemic

The COVID-19 pandemic hit the world with storm in 2020. As a consequence many things changed in the society including our traditional way of learning and it truly challenged the educationists ability to adapt to the situation. Due to social distancing, the pandemic strengthened the necessity for online learning opportunities and virtual education. Many medical schools followed the lockdown procedures with a shift to online and video-based learning. While this might be a temporary shift and end when the pandemic is under control, it could also be the beginning to a new era in teaching. Therefore, we will address certain strategies associated with online learning in this section.

e-Learning or virtual learning has over the past decade in general become a key feature of learning technologies in medical education and even other fields of education. Many business schools for instance offer online Master of Business Administration programs in order to offer flexibility to the individuals work schedule[24]. Multiple studies have shown positive outcomes between e-Learning and medical education[25, 26]. However, they do offer some challenges as well[27]. These barriers mostly included time constraints, poor technical skills, inadequate infrastructure, absence of institutional strategies and support and negative attitudes of all involved[27]. Looking at these barriers, we quickly can find solutions to them including improved educator skills, incentives and reward for the time involved with development and delivery of online content, improved institutional strategies and support and positive attitude amongst all those involved in the development and delivery of online content[27].

First, we will depict the pros and cons with online learning in the medical education context[28]. Advantages:

1. Personalized learning: You can learn at your own time and paste and structure your learning more towards your schedule
2. Long distance learning: you can learn from anywhere: home, coffee shop, library, at your families house etc.
3. Enhancing collaboration and learning: you are able to collaborate and communicate with more people, more institutions and enhance the network of learning
4. Worldwide/statewide exposure: you can take advantage of teaching from other places of the world, schools and professors.
5. Affordable: theoretically, online teaching can be more affordable in the future
6. Improved visualization: through videos, forums in a good educational platform, you can optimize your visualization of your learning
7. Tailor learning towards your strengths: typically, virtual learning includes more than just lectures. It has discussion forums, videos, text etc. If a learning style fits your better, you can focus more on that area than others.
8. Safe time: you theoretically save more time since you don't have to travel to school and back
Disadvantages:
1. Less control over the teaching environment: being an online participant doesn't give you the full control as in a live participant

2. Technical skills: virtual learning requires some technical skills and promptness to work optimally
3. Less real time: you have less real time access and experience in virtual learning
4. Clinical rotations: a full virtual learning system would be very difficult in the medical settings as part of the education requires patient contact. However, some institutions have adopted a virtual sub-internship[29], although the effectiveness of these remains unclear.
5. Laziness: learning from home can make one lazier
6. Loss of bedside teaching and lack of direct patient care
7. Lack of focus and motivation
8. Joint pain, back pain as a result of sitting for hours

ADAPT TO THE NEW SITUATION

In general, knowledge can be obtained in multiple ways. In person, in books, through videos, audiobooks etc. At the end of the day, the primary objective is to learn the necessary knowledge in the field that is within your focus. Thus, even if you are not able to attend classes in person, you can still take advantage of virtual lectures, seminars and discussions or just do self-reading. The foundation of learning will be the same and the faster you just adapt to the situation and accept the circumstances, the better you will do. Moreover, since you theoretically will have more time on your plate, this could be used for your advantage as you can fit in other study session and gain more and faster knowledge than before.

STRUCTURE YOUR TIME

The main thing you have to do when it comes to the virtual sessions is to manage your time well. Since you theoretically may have more time on your plate, you should never overestimate the time you have and structure it as you were going into school. That means that you should set up your own schedule (unless you get one from your school) and follow it religiously. Keep in mind that you will theoretically have more time on your plate since you technically do not have to commute to school back and forth. That means that you can plan in sessions for the time that you would have otherwise been spending on live sessions. Thus, make a schedule, even if your school gives you one, add more things into it so that you are able to fit in more things than usual. This will give you an advantage since you can read more parts in any given day.

GOOD STUDY ENVIRONMENT

It is important that you set up a good study environment even if you are doing virtual learning from home. My recommendation is to view your virtual learning sessions as they were live. Think about what you would have done if you had to go into school and do the same thing. Opening up your laptop in bed and listening half a sleep is not the best way to learn. See this as a "live session" from home. I.e., go back into your own routine. If you took a shower in the morning and grabbed breakfast and coffee before going to school, then do the same thing even if you are sitting at home Infront of your laptop. The more you adapt yourself to the "normal" presence of being in a classroom, the better environment for learning you will provide your brain.

Make sure you sit at a desk with a comfortable chair and good lighting. Make sure you have good earphones to be able to listen optimally. In addition, make sure you have good internet connection so that your session do not lag.

Again, it is all about pretending that you are going into a live session so that you don't get too comfortable. Learning from home can make people lazy if they don't use it the right way.

FOCUS AND REMAIN MOTIVATED

Studies by Machado et al.[30] and Atreya et al.[31] reported the hardships of maintaining focus and concentration whilst sitting in front of a screen. Being in front of the computer all day can make you lose focus. This might not happen to everyone, but it definitely could happen to you. Therefore, it is important to focus on the virtual sessions you have as much as you can. Go back to the session about focus in this book and apply the same tips.

Lee et al[32] found that without academic input, students were more likely to have ineffective learning strategies, poor motivation, and reduced communication. Physical discomfort, such as exhaustion, visual problems, and muscle and joint pain, was also reported with long periods of virtual teaching. Thus, it is important that you take regular breaks, stand up, walk around a bit, and at times even take a bit of fresh air. It is also important just like stated previously in this book that you keep up your motivation, a healthy lifestyle with regular physical activity.

Moreover, it is crucial that you just focus on your teaching and nothing else. As you are likely home alone where no one can see you, there could be tendencies to get distracted doing other things while the virtual session is on. Therefore, I urge you to *not* brows online, check your social media, text message other or do nonrelated activities. Treat each session as someone is watching your back for every activity you are doing.

CATCH UP IN OTHER WAYS

There might be certain virtual activities that doesn't fit your learning style. You might be more of a visual learner or learn best by just reading a text instead of listening. Whatever the case may be, remember that you have a much higher personalized way of learning now with virtual learnings. That means that if a certain session does not teach you much, you still have time to catch up the knowledge in other forms such as reading a book, listening to a video or look up article online. The point is that virtual learning could be very unfamiliar to you but the foundation of learning remains the same. Your key objective is to learn the knowledge in a specific area, and you can still do so in many different ways by yourself or with the help of the virtual learning tools. See what ways that you learn something the best way and focus on that more.

CLINICAL ROTATIONS

Despite the pandemic, medical students have still mostly been able to rotate, at least through their own medical school, in their core rotations. There has however been limitations through travel to other institutions for sub-internships. Nevertheless, how to optimize bedside teaching and direct patient care during a pandemic still remains unclear, but might be a problem that we can control more and more with personal protective equipment being more available, the vaccine for COVID-19 now being available.

Finally, the limited but emerging evidence suggests that virtual teaching is effective, and institutions are working to further develop these resources to improve student engagement and interactivity. Thus, even in an unexpected situation like 2020 brought with the pandemic, if you adapt quickly follow the foundation of learning as depicted in this book, you will most likely learn the sufficient knowledge that is required. Furthermore, the pandemic likely initiated the growth of more improved ways of communication, teaching and technology that will be a reality in the near future[33].

Summary

- Medical school is different from other academic programs with respect to the depth of information you must learn.

- The value of lecture time is that everything gets served to you once before you have to read about it yourself.
- Listening is a skill. You can improve your listening skills through daily practice.
- Focus is a strategic skill that you should invest in improving through practice.
- Good note-taking is important in medical school and another skill that should be mastered. Writing notes makes you remember information from the lecture and allows you to focus better. Assess the different note-taking techniques and adopt the one that works best for you.
- Asking questions is important, but what type of questions to ask is also more important. Don't be afraid of asking questions. In fact, some of the smartest people ask a lot of questions.
- Efficiency is the key to succeeding in medical school, when you need to get many things done in a short time. Being efficient is a function of knowing your priorities. Efficiency is defined as *making the best use of your resources with the least amount of time and effort.*
- Return on investment (ROI) and opportunity cost are two important concepts to apply in your life. ROI is a performance measure used to evaluate the efficiency of an investment or to compare the efficiency of different investments to one another. Opportunity cost is the loss of potential gain from other alternatives when one alternative is chosen.
- Since learning is all about repetition, and since you only remember and grasp a limited amount of information during lectures, reading about the lecture content in advance could help you learn more during class. This should only be done if your time and plan allow for it.

References

1. Andersen SC, Humlum MK, Nandrup AB. Increasing instruction time in school does increase learning. *Proc Natl Acad Sci USA.* 2016;113(27):7481–7484. https://doi.org/10.1073/pnas.1516686113.
2. Tennant K, Toney-Butler TJ. Active Listening. StatPearls.com. https://www.ncbi.nlm.nih.gov/books/NBK442015/. Updated July 7, 2020.
3. Hogan TP, Adlof SM, Alonzo CN. On the importance of listening comprehension. *Int J Speech Lang Pathol.* 2014;16(3):199–207. https://doi.org/10.3109/17549507.2014.904441.
4. Schilling D. 10 Steps to Effective Listening. Forbes.com. https://www.forbes.com/sites/womensmedia/2012/11/09/10-steps-to-effective-listening/#40a290dc3891. Published November 9, 2012.
5. Wadlinger HA, Isaacowitz DM. Fixing our focus: training attention to regulate emotion. *Pers Soc Psychol Rev.* 2011;15(1):75–102. https://doi.org/10.1177/1088868310365565.
6. Moore A, Gruber T, Derose J, Malinowski P. Regular, brief mindfulness meditation practice improves electrophysiological markers of attentional control. *Front Hum Neurosci.* 2012;6:18. https://doi.org/10.3389/fnhum.2012.00018.
7. Mrazek MD, Franklin MS, Phillips DT, Baird B, Schooler JW. Mindfulness training improves working memory capacity and GRE performance while reducing mind wandering. *Psychol Sci.* 2013;24(5):776–781. https://doi.org/10.1177/0956797612459659.
8. Donnelly JE, Hillman CH, Castelli D, et al. Physical activity, fitness, cognitive function, and academic achievement in children: a systematic review. *Med Sci Sports Exerc.* 2016;48(6):1197–1222. https://doi.org/10.1249/MSS.0000000000000901.
9. Adan A. Cognitive performance and dehydration. *J Am Coll Nutr.* 2012;31(2):71–78. https://doi.org/10.1080/07315724.2012.10720011.
10. Allen AP, Smith AP. Effects of chewing gum and time-on-task on alertness and attention. *Nutr Neurosci.* 2012;15(4):176–185. https://doi.org/10.1155/2015/654806.
11. Sharifi P, Rahmati A, Saber M. The effect of note-taking skills training on the achievement motivation in learning on B.A students in Shahid Bahonar University of Kerman and Kerman University of Medical Sciences (Iran). *J Pak Med Assoc.* 2013;63(10):1230–1234.
12. Grahame JA. Digital note-taking: discussion of evidence and best practices. *J Physician Assist Educ.* 2016;27(1):47–50.
13. The Best Note-Taking Methods. GoodNotes. https://medium.goodnotes.com/the-best-note-taking-methods-for-college-students-451f412e264e. Published May 9, 2018.

14. Pohlmann T, Thomas NM. Relearning the Art of Asking Questions. *Harvard Business Review*. https://hbr.org/2015/03/relearning-the-art-of-asking-questions. Published March 27, 2015.

15. Weimer M. The Art of Asking Questions. Faculty Focus. https://www.facultyfocus.com/articles/effective-teaching-strategies/art-asking-questions/. Published May 28, 2014.

16. Fernando J. Return on Investment (ROI). Investopedia. https://www.investopedia.com/terms/r/returnoninvestment.asp. Updated April 27, 2020.

17. Hayes A. Opportunity Cost. Investopedia. https://www.investopedia.com/terms/o/opportunitycost.asp. Updated August 20, 2020.

18. Hann C. The Art of Efficiency: How to Do One Thing at a Time. *Entrepreneur*. https://www.entrepreneur.com/article/226991. Published July 2013.

19. Dewitte S, Schouwenburg HC. Procrastination, temptations, and incentives: the struggle between the present and the future in procrastinators and the punctual. *Eur J Pers*. 2002;16(6):469–489. https://doi.org/10.1002/per.461.

20. Hendriksen E. 5 Ways to Finally Stop Procrastinating. Psychology Today. https://www.psychologytoday.com/us/blog/how-be-yourself/201808/5-ways-finally-stop-procrastinating. Published August 15, 2018.

21. Vanderkam L. *168 Hours: You Have More Time Than You Think*. Portfolio Publishing; 2011.

22. Tracy B. *Eat That Frog!: 21 Great Ways to Stop Procrastinating and Get More Done in Less Time*. Berrett-Koehler Publishing; 2017.

23. Moravec M, Williams A, Aguilar-Roca N, O'Dowd DK. Learn before lecture: a strategy that improves learning outcomes in a large introductory biology class. *CBE Life Sci Educ*. 2010;9(4):473–481. https://doi.org/10.1187/cbe.10-04-0063.

24. AMEE Guide 32. e-Learning in medical education Part 1: Learning, teaching and assessment. In: Ellaway R, Masters K, eds. *Med Teach*. 30(5); *2008:455–473. Jun*.

25. Internet-based learning in the health professions: a meta-analysis. In: Cook DA, Levinson AJ, Garside S, Dupras DM, Erwin PJ, Montori VM, eds. *JAMA*. 300(10); *2008:1181–1196. Sep 10*.

26. Development of e-learning in medical education: 10 years' experience of Korean medical schools. *Kim KJ, Kim G Korean J Med Educ. 2019 Sep; 31(3):205-214*.

27. Barriers and solutions to online learning in medical education - an integrative review. O'Doherty D, Dromey M, Lougheed J, Hannigan A, Last J, McGrath D. *BMC Med Educ. 2018 Jun 7;18(1):130*.

28. EduSys – What is cirtual classrooms? Advantages & Disadvantages. Available at: https://www.edusys.co/blog/what-is-virtual-classroom.

29. Yale School of Medicine, plastic surgery virtual sub-*internships: https://medicine.yale.edu/surgery/plastics/education/medstudents/*.

30. Machado R, Bonan P, Perez DED, Martelli D, Martelli-Júnior H. I am having trouble keeping up with virtual teaching activities: Reflections in the COVID-19 era. In: *Clinics (Sao Paulo). 75; 2020:e1945*. https://doi.org/10.6061/clinics/2020/e1945.

31. Atreya A, Acharya J. Distant virtual medical education during COVID-19: Half a loaf of bread. *Clin Teach*. 2020 Jun 18;17(4):418–419. https://doi.org/10.1111/tct.13185.

32. Lee I, Koh H, Lai S, Hwang N. Academic coaching of medical students during the COVID-19 pandemic. *Med Educ*. 2020 Jun;(12). https://doi.org/10.1111/medu.14272.

33. Wilcha RJ. Effectiveness of Virtual Medical Teaching During the COVID-19 Crisis: Systematic Review. *JMIR Med Educ*. 2020 Nov 18;6(2):e20963. https://doi.org/10.2196/20963. PMID: 33106227; PMCID: PMC7682786.

CHAPTER 9

Mentors in Medical School

I think a role model is a mentor—someone you see on a daily basis, and you learn from them.
—Denzel Washington

A mentor is someone who is willing to give you advice that isn't in the best interest for them. It takes a real mentor to put you first.
—Caroline Ghosn

Anyone who has been successful and has knowledge to share is a potential mentor.
—Ory Okolloh

CHAPTER OUTLINE

Introduction

I hung up the phone without saying goodbye.

My mentor called me back right away and asked, "What's wrong, Raman? You never hang up like that."

"I'm tired," I answered. "I've got all these deadlines and projects, I'm writing my new book, working on two research manuscripts, and have my clinical exam coming up in one week, et cetera."

"Okay. That's not anything you haven't done before," he said.

"At the same time, I feel like people are acting different towards me, and it stresses me out because I don't know why," I continued.

"Raman, let me ask you: Have you ever doubted yourself? Ever cried at night because of pain? Ever thought you're going crazy? Ever thought about how so-and-so is not calling anymore? Ever wondered why people start hating you and bugging you for no reason? Ever thought about giving up?"

"Yes!" I said, perking up. "All of the above!"

"Okay, let me tell you the inevitabilities of success since I don't think you understand them at this juncture in your life:

"You will feel pain. You will cry 100 times. You will doubt yourself 1000 times. You *will* lose friends. People *will* hate you for no reason. You *will* think you're going crazy. And you *will* come close to talking yourself out of it many times. Understand, this is all just a part of the process! However, you know what the best part is? It'll all be worth it one day. Focus."

This is a conversation that unfolded one October night during my time as a medical student. My mentor guided me, honestly advised me, and motivated me to keep going even though things felt impossibly hard in that moment. If you've been paying attention, then this pep talk should sound familiar to you. (See Chapter 2 for a reminder.)

Mentors

At this stage of your life, if you're lucky, you may already have found a mentor. A mentor is a friend, role model, or a person who guides someone less experienced by building trust and modeling positive behaviors[1]. Basically, a mentor is an experienced and trusted advisor. A mentor shares information about their own career path and provides guidance, emotional support, and motivation[1]. They will help you to set your goals, discuss them, explore different career paths, identify resources, and even help you network.

Why Mentorship in Medical School is Important

As a student thinking about a career in medicine or already enrolled in medical school, you are likely smart and ambitious and used to figuring things out for yourself. This is the reason why you are where you are today. Many successful people figure out the path to success on their own, often through trial and error. Sooner or later (often later), we come upon a system that works for us and ultimately succeed in what we would like to do. And while this is a common path to follow, the reality is that things can happen faster and more efficiently if you are guided by someone more experienced who has already done it before you. That person has already taken the path that you are trying to take and knows the mistakes they made. As a result, they can advise you to avoid the mistakes they made and to do the things that they should have done[2,3].

Regardless of how smart you are, your lack of experience means that you may not always know exactly what should be done and how and in what time frame. While you might figure it out for yourself eventually, you might end up wasting a lot of time, start too late, or progress far slower than you'd like.

I will never forget the day when one of my third-year medical students saw a plastic surgery case for the first time. She had felt so inspired that she started crying afterward. When I asked her what was wrong, she said that she had finally found what she liked but that it was too late to match into such a highly competitive field like plastic surgery. Had she found a mentor earlier to help her explore different options, she might have found herself in a different situation that day[2,3].

Just like a real-life mentor, this book is also intended to work as your "mentor," guiding you to a successful path in medical school. By learning about trial and error, science-based evidence, and strategies that have worked (and not worked), you are positioning yourself to be at a competitive advantage compared with those who will never read this book. You will learn what to do and what not do. You will learn all the study techniques that have worked for thousands and given them a path to success, which will make you much better prepared than others.

Someone out there has already done the work you are planning on doing. They have already attempted the trial-and-error approach. They know all about the obstacles, the shortcuts, the tactics, and the strategies. They know what to avoid and what opportunities to pursue.

Imagine for a moment that you are standing in an operating room, wearing your surgical scrubs. A patient is lying on the operating table. Someone hands you a scalpel. With zero preparation or training, do you think you could successfully perform an operation by figuring out all the techniques on your own? Now, imagine that a capable mentor has taught you what to do first, and you have practiced many times under their watchful eye. How prepared do you feel now? That is the gift of a mentor: they know what things to focus on (and when) and what things not to waste your time on. You know time is limited. So the better prepared you are by someone who can guide you through the process, the better your chances of success[2,3].

The advantages of mentors are as follows[4,5]:

1. **Knowledge.** Mentors provide knowledge and information. A mentor will not only offer you their insight about a specific field, but they can also show you how it's done and involve you in it. As Benjamin Franklin said, "Tell me and I forget; teach me and I may remember; involve me and I learn." Guided by a mentor from the start, you will run into a wealth of knowledge that will get you up to speed much faster.

2. **Personal development.** A mentor can see where you need to improve. A good mentor will be honest with you and tell it like it is. If you are interested in a specific field, they will tell you what is required and the things you need to do in order to reach your goal. They will provide constructive criticism that will help you see things in yourself that you cannot see. George Lucas once said, "Mentors have a way of seeing more of our faults than we would like. It's the only way we grow."

3. **Motivation and inspiration.** One of the main reasons I chose plastic surgery as a specialty was because I had a great mentor in medical school who was a plastic surgeon and who inspired me tremendously. Mentors are there to motivate you to be better, push harder, and put in more effort. They will guide you and inspire you to do the right things. They have likely experienced many hardships on their own career paths and can therefore share important lessons with you.

4. **Trusted advisors.** In the world of medicine, it can be difficult to know whom to trust. Since a mentor is typically an objective third party with no personal stake in your success or failure, they usually have your best interests at heart. Therefore, you can usually fully trust a mentor and reveal your deepest concerns and insecurities.

5. **Networking.** Connections are key in any field, but especially in medical school. Your desired specialty could be highly competitive. If your mentor knows important people in that field, it could help you tremendously with getting interviews and even securing a residency position. I cannot count the number of times that people I know have matched into residency positions thanks to their connections.

6. **Research.** Nowadays, a successful applicant ideally has a research background and publications on their CV. A mentor in the medical field could connect you to research opportunities that give you the chance to publish in scientific journals and boost your CV.

7. **Trial and error.** Starting medical school, acing your exams, doing well on your rotations, and matching into a residency program is challenging enough, so if you can skip doing things the hard way, why wouldn't you? A mentor has been there, right where you currently are, and has made plenty of mistakes that they can now tell you about. This is not the time for experimentation through trial and error. A mentor can help you avoid the potentially devastating effects of your not knowing.

8. **Free advice.** Mentors are free, which makes them literally priceless. A mentor does not do things for money. Instead, they are driven by the satisfaction of helping another, of paying it forward from a similar experience they had when starting on their path to success. Therefore, you will never owe them anything or pay them money to get their advice. They are there for your benefit without your needing to spend a dime.

How to Find a Mentor

Mentors are everywhere. It could be one of your teachers, one of your professors, one of your supervisors, or someone else that inspired you in some way. The main thing is to reach out to them.

Talk to them, email them, or even call them. Once you find a role model or someone that you look up to, you need to take the initiative. Mentors will not seek you out. You have to actively search for them and contact them. This is an investment that will be worth spending time on because it could pay off big time. If you already have someone in mind, Google them to learn more about them and to get their contact information. Then write to them. If you have not already found a potential mentor, then I encourage you to actively seek one. Be open to it during your classes, interactions with people during your rotations, and so on. Think about who inspired you and arrange to meet with that person[6].

Once you have found a mentor, you need to maintain the relationship. Most mentors are busy. They typically have a number of commitments—running their own practice, maintaining their laboratory, or serving as the chair or dean of a department. Therefore, you need to be proactive and use your time (and their time) wisely. Email them and set up monthly check-ins and meetings and be flexible and try to accommodate their schedule. If they are still too busy to be your mentor at the moment, be creative and try to come up with a way you can meet them in person.

Once you do meet in person, be honest with them about your goals and aspirations. Tell them what you want to get out of a mentorship and show them who you are. Remember to be kind, respectful, and very appreciative of their time. Politeness and gratitude are extremely important.

Finally, remember that most mentors were likely once in your shoes and had *their* own mentor. Now, they are in a position to pay it forward. Thus, the best way to repay a mentor is to pay it forward yourself one day. Once you reach your goals, or wherever you are in your career, there is someone who can benefit from your advice. Not only does it offer you the opportunity to give back, you will also receive a lot of satisfaction in return.

Summary

- A mentor is a friend, role model, or a person who guides someone less experienced by building trust and modeling positive behaviors. A mentor is an experienced and trusted advisor.
- A mentor has walked the road you are walking today and can help to guide you and avoid the pitfalls.
- A mentor can support you in many ways, both personally and professionally. They can help you with networking, research connections, motivation, and inspiration. And the best thing about mentorship is that it is totally free.
- Actively search for a mentor. Having a good mentor can pay off big time. Once you find a potential mentor, contact them, maintain the relationship, and then pay it forward when you are in a position to do so.

References

1. Mentor. Cambridge Dictionary. https://dictionary.cambridge.org/us/dictionary/english/mentor. Accessed September 17, 2020.
2. Taherian K, Shekarchian M. Mentoring for doctors: do its benefits outweigh its disadvantages? *Med Teach.* 2008;30(4):e95–e99. https://doi.org/10.1080/01421590801929968.
3. Burgess A, van Diggele C, Mellis C. Mentorship in the health professions: a review. *Clin Teach.* 2018;15(3):197–202. https://doi.org/10.1111/tct.12756.
4. Lusinski N. 7 Reasons to Get a Career Mentor, Even if You Love Your Job. Bustle.com. https://www.bustle.com/p/7-benefits-of-having-a-career-mentor-even-if-you-love-your-job-2842979. Published January 26, 2018.

5. Brushfield R. 21 Benefits of Getting a Mentor. *The Telegraph*. November 30, 2012. https://jobs.telegraph.co.uk/article/21-benefits-of-getting-a-mentor/.
6. Darvers B. Physician Mentorship: Why it's Important, and How to Find and Sustain Relationships. *The New England Journal of Medicine* Career Center website. https://www.nejmcareercenter.org/article/physician-mentorship-why-it-s-important-and-how-to-find-and-sustain-relationships-/. Published February 28, 2018.

CHAPTER 10

Strategies with Classmates

Surround yourself with good people; surround yourself with positivity and people who are going to challenge you to make you better.
—Ali Krieger

Surround yourself with only people who are going to lift you higher.
—Oprah Winfrey

Introduction

You are greatly affected by people in your environment, far more than you think. Social relationships are essential for your survival and tend to affect your thoughts, feelings, and behaviors. During your medical school years, you will meet many people, some of whom you will have closer contact with than others. It is important to think about who you are networking and socializing with because it can often affect your choices and performance in life.

How Others Affect You

Success in medical school and in life is mainly related to you, the choices you make, and the amount of work hard you put in. However, your success is also related to the people you spend your time with. Have you ever wondered how similar groups of people who all hang out together achieve similar levels of success? Whether this is a low or high level of success, the members of a group influence each other and most end up on similar paths[1–3].

If you end up with a group of students who are high achievers, enjoy school, study hard, and believe in the importance of success, you will most likely be influenced to do the same. Therefore, one of the keys to a successful medical school strategy is to spend time with the right people. From the very beginning, it is vitally important to consider whom you choose to spend most of these years with so that you get the right kind of influence[1–3].

In every class, students can be ranked according to their grades. There will always be some students who are better than others. The ranking of students means that they will have different overall GPAs and levels of success by graduation. That is why some students end up graduating top of their class while others do not. Typically, smarter students congregate with each other, a pattern you see in many fields, not just in medical school.

Therefore, if you want to succeed in medical school, you should be strategic about whom you spend time with. Do your best to identify these high achievers early on. Make a plan to join up with other ambitious groups of students, and try to choose your study partners carefully. As the saying goes, "If you are the smartest person in the room, you are in the wrong room." You need to surround yourself with people who are smarter than you or are at least at the same level of intelligence, ambition, and motivation. Then you will constantly develop yourself to become a better version of yourself and be more motivated to study hard[1-3].

From now on, try to socialize and join a circle of smart, hard-working people. It will allow you to constantly grow and achieve higher levels of success in medical school. If you hang out with the wrong crowd, then your progress and development will be hampered and, in some cases, lead to poorer life choices. If you hang out with lazy people, then there is a risk that you will also become lazier. If you hang out with those who want to party, skip class, and avoid studying, there is a greater chance that they will influence you to do the same. Whatever activities your social group engages in, you will also most likely do the same. I have seen this pattern with my own eyes, with my own classmates, through all my years of school. The same patterns held true even when I did my Master of Business Administration and then my executive Master of Healthcare Leadership, programs in which the average age was much higher than mine. Therefore, think strategically about the people who can most benefit you and keep all others at a distance[1-3].

When to Compare Yourself to Others

We humans tend to compare ourselves to others, from movie stars to our friends. This is a natural behavior that can actually be beneficial if you do it with care. Although many argue that you should compare yourself only to yourself and compete only with yourself, it is in fact healthy to know where you are in relation to others. This comparison could serve as a baseline whereby you can intermittently check whether you are moving ahead.

If you discover that you rank much higher than others in terms of grades, scores, and evaluations, then you know that you are doing something right and that you should continue the same way. However, even if this is the case, I encourage you to never slow down just because you are scoring higher than others. Keep moving towards your goals at the same pace. Regular comparison to others can serve as a good mental alarm: if you notice yourself starting to slip or someone quickly approaching your level, let it serve as a warning to put in some more effort. Conversely, if you notice that you are far behind others in your grades, scores, or evaluations, let it serve as fuel to reevaluate your strategy and work harder. Don't feel bad—instead, inspire yourself by the success and ambitions of others and try to do what they are doing to achieve their level of success.

Some will argue that you should never compare yourself to others. I believe that people make this argument because they do not want you to be disappointed or feel bad if others are more accomplished than you. My counterargument is that you likely compare yourself with others automatically, but without reflecting on it or allowing it to affect you negatively. The effect of comparison depends on how you see the situation. You could feel disappointed in yourself or you could see it as inspiration and a teachable moment; I encourage you to do the latter. Looking at others' success is not something that should make you feel bad, but instead should be used as inspiration to do the same, using the tools they used. In business, we call it modeling, whereby one business looks at other successful businesses in order to do a particular thing just as well, if not better.

In addition, a business will look at what mistakes competitors have made and avoid these mistakes themselves. So don't be afraid to look at others who have been more successful than you have: simply determine how they behaved so that you can learn from and emulate them.

Group Assignments

In medical school, you will have group assignments or tasks to perform with other students. Sometimes you get to pick the students in your group, sometimes you don't. When you do get to select your group, it will be important that you have already started orienting yourself to find friends in class who have the same goals and values as you do. It is always easier to perform well if you have competent support along the way. Ambitious, generous students can inspire you personally, and together you can create a group that collaborates well together and inspires each other to do better.

Remember that in the beginning, when you are starting a new class, you will have no idea which students are ambitious or not, who will stick around in the program or not. In the beginning, everyone is similarly motivated, which makes it even more difficult to be selective. But the dust usually clears after the first couple of tests. Of those students who received good scores, grades, or evaluations in the beginning, only some will continue to prove themselves to be energetic, intelligent, and ambitious. You will want to seek partners for group assignments who show most or all of these qualities, as these students will probably be able to maintain the same level of success and help you achieve better results.

You can also take the time to notice who the more talented students are by their way of asking and answering questions and their ability to discuss various topics in class. A student's engagement in the classroom or during rotations can give clues about their intelligence. The talented students will usually want to appear better, which is noticeable early on. These are people you should spend your time studying with. Many of the projects and assignments you did in high school were done in groups. Doing group work with talented students also gives you the opportunity to learn things from others. When you read part of someone's work, notice all the phrases and terms they have used, and mimic that for your future work. If you work with talented people, you will soon be up to their level. However, if you work with students who are not smart, hard-working, and ambitious, then you will always be uncertain about whether their work is good or not. In addition, there is a risk that others will not commit to doing their part.

You Are Allowed to Choose Whom You Work With

People sometimes ask me, "Isn't it wrong to choose your classmates?" The answer to that question is no. It's absolutely not wrong. Just as you choose your regular friends in your leisure time according to your particular social needs, or your spouse or partner based on your unique criteria, you can also choose classmates in alignment with your future goals. Medical school is not a club where you are meant to socialize with people for fun. It is a serious full-time job that will determine your future. In the business world, professionals choose to socialize and network with the smartest, best, and most skilled people all the time, simply because it is how their own businesses develop for the better.

Being a bad student is a conscious choice that some people make. There are no excuses. Anyone could become a good student if they put in the effort. Thus, if students choose not to work hard in medical school, they must blame themselves for both their poor grades and their failures. If you meet a person with good qualities who you want to socialize with, you should openly share that you are aiming to do well and that collaborating together might be a good fit and benefit both. Please note that you are the sole person responsible for your success. But if you get help along the way from better and smarter students, it can never hurt; on the contrary, it can only benefit you, and this is another important factor to success in your medical career.

Remember also that the benefits of such relationships go both ways: choosing smarter people to hang out and work with does not mean that you can do poor work. Just the opposite: you should do your utmost to bring the most value you can to the group and the work you do. Hard work and high value are always noticed, and so is the opposite. People will quickly notice whether or not you're contributing well to something; you don't want to end up in a situation where others want to avoid working with *you* because they don't believe in your abilities or work ethic. Always work hard. Bring the greatest value you can at all times, and show people that you are an asset to the group.

Act Like and Be the Smartest Student in the Class

You should always show that you want to be the best in the class. Make everyone aware that you want to get the best grades and graduate top of your class. Show no weaknesses, and illustrate that you are a responsible student. Show yourself to be a person who works hard and is motivated to achieve your goals. When you do, then others who are just as intelligent and ambitious will gather around *you* and want to socialize with *you*. That way *you* don't have to find the smarter people, *they* will find you[4,5].

I never needed to find smart classmates to hang out with; they found me instead. The truth was that both highly skilled and less skilled students approached me and wanted to hang out, after they realized that I was performing well. But I chose to spend time with only people who could help me and contribute to my success just as I could theirs. If, however, I had not shown myself to be a hard worker, I can promise you that not many would have wanted to spend time with me either. This is a natural instinct. Very few people want to be with someone who is a low performer and doesn't care about the things that are important to their future. We all want to surround ourselves with strong, hard-working, ambitious people so that we can adopt these skills[4,5].

The students I chose to do group assignments with or to study with were very smart and worked hard. They were people who really helped me when I needed it. Only later did I truly understand the value they brought me, which is why I am teaching you the same now. Therefore, show everyone that you are smart, skilled, and capable of learning everything in an excellent way. You will then be liked by others, attract other successful students, and work well with others. By acting like and being the smartest person in the class, you will soon see that other students will come up to you to ask you questions. They will want your help as well as your opinions on topics that were raised. If you come across as an intelligent person, you will also get a lot of attention in class. Your thoughts will be valued, and your voice will be heard and expected by everyone during each discussion. Teachers will also see and notice your ambition, which will further increase your status and evaluations in class[4-6].

Summary

- You are greatly influenced by the people around you. Therefore, surround yourself with ambitious classmates who are intelligent and have the same work ethic that you do. This will help you, develop you, and galvanize your path toward success in medical school.
- Compare yourself with your peers from time to time to see where you are in relation to them. This way you can get an idea of whether you need to move into a higher gear or if the speed you are driving at right now is just right.
- You will do many group assignments in school. If you have talented and ambitious students to do group assignments with, you will work together to do an even better job. Moreover, you do not run the risk of having to sit and do most of the work yourself, which can happen if your peers do not do their part.

- Strive to always be the best student in the class and make a point of showing it. Then, other excellent students will approach you and want to hang out with you. In this way, you can be selective about the people you want to hang out with and do group assignments with. This also gives you higher status in the class and makes you a valued student in all situations.

References

1. Tomé G, Matos M, Simões C, Diniz JA, Camacho I. How can peer group influence the behavior of adolescents: explanatory model. *Glob J Health Sci.* 2012;4(2):26–35. https://doi.org/10.5539/gjhs.v4n2p26.
2. Flashman J. Academic achievement and its impact on friend dynamics. *Sociol Educ.* 2012;85(1):61–80. https://doi.org/10.1177/0038040711417014.
3. Moussaïd M, Kämmer JE, Analytis PP, Neth H. Social influence and the collective dynamics of opinion formation. *PLoS One.* 2013;8(11):e78433. https://doi.org/10.1371/journal.pone.0078433.
4. Bergagna E, Tartaglia S. Self-esteem, social comparison, and Facebook use. *Eur J Psychol.* 2018;14(4):831–845. https://doi.org/10.5964/ejop.v14i4.1592.
5. Metzler A, Scheithauer H. The long-term benefits of positive self-presentation via profile pictures, number of friends and the initiation of relationships on Facebook for adolescents' self-esteem and the initiation of offline relationships. *Front Psychol.* 2017;8:1981. https://doi.org/10.3389/fpsyg.2017.01981.
6. Booth MZ, Gerard JM. Self-esteem and academic achievement: a comparative study of adolescent students in England and the United States. *Compare.* 2011;41(5):629–648. https://doi.org/10.1080/030579 25.2011.566688.

CHAPTER 11

Memorization and Learning Techniques

Be stubborn about your goals and flexible about your methods.
—Unknown

*Yesterday I was clever, so I changed the world. Today I am wise,
so I am changing myself.*
—Rumi

Introduction

A good memory will make your study time far more effective. In college and medical school, there are many things that you will need to memorize and remember, not just to do well on your exams but also to excel in your future career as a physician. There is an enormous amount of information that you need to process and learn in every course. Therefore, if you have a good baseline memory, it will help you with your studies. However, the strength of memory varies from person to person.

Some people can read a text twice and remember 90% of the content, while others need to read the same text 10 times to remember the same amount of information. Although you might process information differently from your neighbour and might have a weaker memory, it is possible to improve your memory through different memorization strategies.

I have spent the majority of my life in school. I currently hold a medical degree, a Master of Business and Administration degree, and an executive Master of Healthcare Leadership degree. Since high school I have graduated from all my degrees with a 4.0 grade point average (GPA). This means that I have never received a B in a single course—not in high school, nor in medical school or either of my master's programs. You may think that I'm one of the smartest people on the planet. While I am intelligent, my performance in school—learning new things, remembering them, and getting good grades—had far more to do with learning methods, study techniques, and motivation than pure intelligence. However, one of the factors that will help you succeed in school is having a good baseline memory. If you would not describe yourself as having a good memory, do not panic. This chapters presents different memorization techniques that are designed to improve your learning and memory[1-3].

The Brain and Memory

The brain is the most complex and fascinating organ in the human body. It consists of a sophisticated network of nerve cells that integrate in ways we do not yet fully understand[4]. How our memory works is equally fascinating. Right now, as you are reading this text, your brain is processing each letter, word, and sentence and then tries to make meaning out of the text as well as incorporate it into your memory[4]. This process is responsible for why you are able to remember the names of your friends, books that you have read, dishes that you have eaten, and so on.

Two Forms of Knowledge

In medical school, the knowledge that you will acquire can be divided into two categories: procedural knowledge and factual knowledge. Procedural knowledge is self-explanatory. It consists of all the practical parts of your medical education: how to suture, how to draw blood, how to insert a central line[5]. Factual knowledge is all the theoretical knowledge that you will learn, such as the physiology of the heart, the anatomy of the brain, and how sepsis occurs. Factual knowledge consists of "what", "how," and "why" information[5].

Procedural knowledge can be learned through practice. This is why you may have heard that even a monkey could potentially perform an operation if they did the same procedure enough times. However, factual knowledge—which makes up the majority of the content in medical school—is more difficult to learn, as it requires a lot of repetition, reading, testing, and summarizing. It is also the knowledge that most students feel stressed and overwhelmed by, since the volume of information to learn is massive[6]. Unfortunately, most schools do not teach students *how* to learn *before* they actually start teaching students the content[7]. And that is precisely the role of this book: to teach you how to learn *before* you are required to absorb a seemingly impossible amount of information.

How You Learn Factual Knowledge

Think about how you learn something the best way. Take type 1 diabetes for instance. You learn about what type 1 diabetes is as well as its symptoms, pathophysiology, incidence, treatment, and complications. You learn this knowledge through lectures, reading about it, building mnemonics, and then repeating the information. Your learning will have been successful when you are able to recall what diabetes is, how many new diagnoses we have per year, what the treatments and complications are, and so on. You build associations in your brain and categorize this knowledge in the spectrum of diseases. Simply put, you learn by repeating things many times and in different ways[8]. Repetition is the core technique for building knowledge. The more you repeat something, the more ingrained it becomes. Through repetition, the brain can more easily remember and recall knowledge whenever you need it. Thus, repetition is the key to learning factual knowledge. Your repetitions can involve listening to a lecture first, reading the information in your textbook, reviewing your notes, or listening to a recording. Knowledge is stored in the memory by repeatedly taking in the same information many times, preferably in different ways[8].

Why You Forget

Although the brain is designed for information storage and retrieval, why is it that you still forget things? Forgetting is the process by which you lose or are not able to retrieve information stored in your memory, even though the information has been deposited. For instance, you might forget what the incidence of type 1 diabetes is or what its main complications are.

Hermann Ebbinghaus, a German psychologist, hypothesized that the process of forgetting follows a curve, an observation he made after experimenting with the memorization of nonsense syllables and subsequent testing of the retention of these syllables[8]. Consequently, the memorization of new information follows a time curve: when the information is not repeated in one way or another, the neurological pathways that keep signaling for that specific information grow weaker and then fade away. Thus, any new factual knowledge that you acquire is destined to be forgotten if it is not repeated (i.e., if you learn it only once).

Furthermore, the more complex a subject is, the more often it needs to be repeated to be learned. And that complexity is individual: learning about type 1 diabetes may be straightforward for some and difficult for others. Many students get frustrated when they read things once or twice and then cannot recall the information. Learning about new subjects and memorizing a lot of information takes time and is simply the way the brain is designed—a big part of learning is repetition. More complex subjects in particular require several rounds of repetition to be learned effectively for later recall; the key is to not allow yourself to get frustrated while learning[9].

Can You Improve Your Memory?

The simple answer is yes. Many studies have shown that memory can be improved regardless of what your baseline is. One of my favorite studies was done by a Swedish psychologist who published his results in *Science*. Ericsson and colleagues recruited undergraduate students with average memory skills and intelligence and asked them to recall a sequence of random digits that were given to them at the rate of one digit per second[10]. In the beginning, they could only recall around seven numbers in a row. He then asked them to practice this sequence of numbers for 1 hour a day, 3 to 5 times per week. After about 20 months of practice, the students could recall a sequence of nearly 80 digits. These and many other studies confirm that your memory can be improved with practice[10].

Practice has a powerful effect on memorization or repetition for knowledge retention. Without practice, you will quickly lose the information you learned according to Ebbinghaus' forgetting curve. However, with practice, your memory can be trained, the same way muscles are trained at the gym.

Remember, You Already Have a Decent Memory

Most people are of average intelligence. This conclusion is obvious if you are familiar with the normal distribution of intelligence and IQ. Consequently, with average intelligence, you should already have a decent memory. If others seem to have a better memory than you, it is usually due to the following three things:

1. **Genetics:** Genetics plays a role in our intelligence, the same way it does our height, memory, and other traits.
2. **Practice:** Some students have practiced and studied hard for many years. With more practice comes better memorization and recall of information.
3. **Belief in your abilities:** For this final point, I will give you a personal example, but you can find dozens of studies and books on the placebo effect and the power of belief. If you believe you can do something, such as improving your learning and memorization skills, then you are more likely to be successful in your efforts.

MY FRIEND MARIAM

Back in high school, I had a friend—let's call her Mariam (not her real name)—who said she was really good at remembering numbers. She could easily remember people's phone numbers, their ages, the years they were born, and other strings of numbers. In contrast, she would always tell everyone that she had a terrible memory for anything that did not relate to numbers.

One day, after hearing Mariam make this claim for the hundredth time, I told her that this could not possibly be true. I bluntly asked her how was it that she could be so good at remembering digits and so bad at remembering everything else, since the memory is pretty much the same regardless of what information is given to it.

She then said something that I will never forget: "Raman, I don't know what it is, but when it comes to numbers I am so confident about it, and I am known to be good at it, so when a sequence of numbers or digits comes up, I get so focused and concentrate on it so much that I remember it."

At that moment, I understood that learning is likely related to how confident you are in yourself, and that your belief system plays a role in your ability to remember things.

I challenged Mariam to put as much focus and energy into remembering things other than just numbers, such as a text, to see whether she could remember that just as well. After only 2 weeks, she called me to say that she had received an A on a course in social science, in which there were massive texts to understand and memorize. Today, Mariam is a successful entrepreneur and has two master's degrees under her belt.

As you can see from this real-life example, memory is linked to your belief system. What changed for Mariam? Nothing more than the fact that she began to believe that her memory for other things could be just as good as her memory for numbers. And that belief carried her far.

Confucius, a Chinese philosopher, once said, "He who thinks he can and he who thinks that he cannot, are both usually right."

I strongly believe in this quote because life really does play out that way. If you believe you are going to be good at something or able to do something well, you will most likely be able to. Conversely, if you do not think, at baseline, that you will be able to achieve something, such as memorizing information, you will likely not be good at it.

Thus, confidence in your capability to learn new things will play a big role in your success as a student and beyond. You must believe that you are capable of learning new information and learning it well. From today onward, you should have this attitude whenever you open your books. Be patient with yourself and understand that learning and memorization take practice. Such an attitude will help you along the way, as will confidence in yourself and your beliefs about what you can and cannot do.

Exercises to Strengthen Your Memory and Ability to Learn

Research has shown that your memory improves when you use effective memorization techniques[1-4]. The memory is like a muscle in the body—if you work it out regularly, it will be much stronger (Figure 11.1). But just like a physical workout, it's important to build your memory

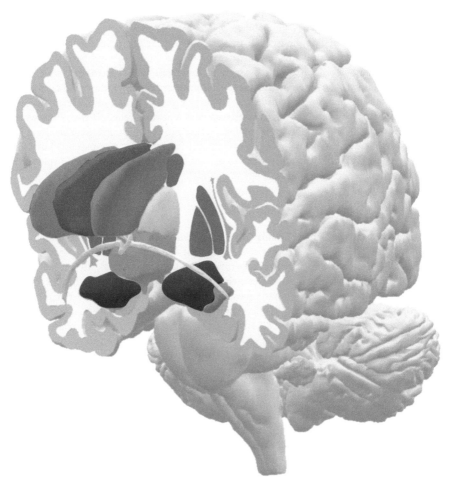

Fig. 11.1 Brain. (Reused with permission from Vanderah T, Gould D. *Nolte's The Human Brain*, 8th ed. Elsevier; 2020. Figure 23.1.)

"muscles" the right way. The methods that follow are effective and based on scientific evidence and the experiences of many students.

REPETITION: THE FOUNDATION OF THE TECHNIQUES

Imagine that you are standing before a field of thick grass that reaches up to your head and that you need to walk through this grass to get to the other side. The first time you walk through the grass, it will be rather slow and laborious, as you will have to push down the tall grass every step of the way. It will also be difficult to find your path because the grass will block your line of sight. Thus, you will exert a lot of energy to cross the field the first time. But with some struggle and hard work, you will ultimately reach your goal.

Now, imagine that you want to walk through the grass along the same path a second time. It will be much easier for a few reasons. First, you have taken this path once already, so you can somewhat recognize it. Second, the thick and tall grass is not as high and dense anymore, and therefore you can get through it more easily. Third, it will require less energy, which also gives a subjective feeling of ease.

Your brain contains a much more complex network of cells than is illustrated by a path through tall grass[4], but this simple analogy shows how a memory is created. When you read something for the first time, you are building the path for that memory for the first time. The more you repeat that information, the more well-worn that path becomes, and the easier it will be for the signals to travel along this path in order to create that memory and recall the information.

The foundation of many memory techniques is repetition. However, the techniques differ in the way you repeat them: how you do it, how frequently you do it, and so on. It's important to know exactly how much time you need in between each repetition round. If you repeat with too short spaces, then you are just wasting your time because you already remember it well, and if you repeat it with too much time apart, then you have already forgotten the information. Thus, balance is one of the key factors and one of the most important things in learning is to find your optimal time interval between the repetitions.

UNDERSTANDING

The best way to remember something is to fully understand it[11]. Understanding is not a memory technique in itself but rather something that should be the primary goal for all of your learning. While certain information is difficult to understand (e.g., the names of drugs, muscles, and bones), there are principles behind the way they are named. In fact, much of the terminology used in medicine has a meaning behind it, and learning these naming principles will facilitate your learning. Understanding these principles first—as opposed to just memorizing the names of things—will allow you to better understand and retain the names of, to use our example, drugs, muscles, and bones. Therefore, I urge you to try to understand to the best of your ability everything you are learning in each course. But understanding and recalling information will also require you to remember it, and that is why I will also teach you memorization techniques.

ASSOCIATION

One of the most efficient ways to remember something is through association. If you associate information with things you already know, for instance, your chances of remembering the new information will increase. If you forget the newly acquired knowledge, you can remember what you had associated it with, which is already stored in your long-term memory, and this will help you to remember the new information. If I tell you to remember the sequence 29035 it could be difficult to remember on its own. However, if I tell you that 29035 is how tall Mount Everest is in feet, then you have now associated that number with something you are already familiar with, which will help you remember[11].

An even longer sequence of digits, such as 29035090531, can be even more difficult to remember. However, if I split the numbers up and associate each of the parts with something I already know, it would make it easier to remember the entire number. For instance, I could associate 29035 with the height of Mount Everest, 0905 with the month and day I was born, and 31 with the age of my best friend. If at some point I forget the total sequence of numbers, then I can ask myself:

1. How tall is Mount Everest?
2. What month and day was I born?
3. How old is my best friend?

With the association technique, I want you to use your imagination to the fullest. The weirder and funnier, in fact, the better. You can use this for any type of knowledge you would like to memorize just by being creative. The names of nerves, muscles, arteries, and veins are just a few aspects of human anatomy that this technique could be useful for.

CHUNKING

It is easier to memorize small amounts of information than large amounts. With chunking, you break up a large list of information into smaller chunks. For instance, you can group information into categories. Let's say you want to memorize a list of medications. You can start by chunking the medications into different categories, such as antiviral, antibacterial, and antifungal. From there, you can list all the different medications within each group. You can break it down into even smaller chunks by further dividing each category into subcategories. For antibiotics, you can chunk them into penicillin, cephalosporins, and fluoroquinolones and then name each drug in each subcategory.

You also can chunk images. Take the citric acid cycle for instance. Breaking it down into eight parts and learning each part individually simplifies the learning process and is easier than trying to learn the entire cycle at once[12].

VISUALIZATION

You tend to learn something better when you visualize it. I use this technique whenever I want to remember where I put my keys. I visualize the setting or place where I could have last placed the keys, and it always makes me remember where I actually put them. In anatomy, for instance, it is much easier to learn the information by first conceptualizing it rather than just learning the terms. This is why we have anatomy dissection labs in medical school. The same goes with other courses such as pharmacology. If you want to remember the pharmacokinetics of a particular drug, try to visualize where the drug is metabolized, which paths in the body it takes, and which cell it affects and it will be easier to remember. Some students like to draw their own diagrams. Although this could be time-consuming, if you enjoy drawing then it might help you remember things more efficiently (Figure 11.2). You can also use your imagination here and create images in your brain that are illogical, irrational, or emotional. Whatever works for you. The sky's the limit of what you can imagine[11].

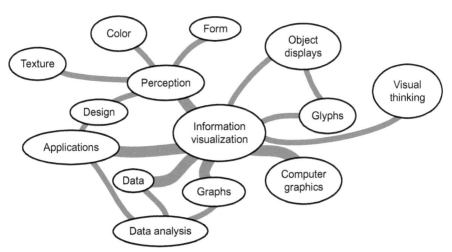

Fig. 11.2 A mind map surrounding the concept of information visualization. Only a few of the possible links are shown. (Reused with permission from Ware C. *Information Visualization: Perception for Design*, 4th ed. Elsevier; 2020. Figure 8.20.)

FLASHCARDS

Flashcards are used by many students. They typically consist of a question on one side of the card and the answer on the other side. You pick up a card, read the question, and try to answer it, then read the answer to check whether you were right. Flashcards help with memorization in many ways. First, when you are actively trying to answer a question, you are forced to recall the memory that was created through your learning. Second, when you read the answer, it adds a round of repetition. Third, reading the answer to a question helps you to associate that knowledge with that question, which could further help you when that question shows up on your exam. Fourth, when you do not know the answer, it is right there for you to learn it[11].

RETRIEVAL PRACTICE

This method involves describing to yourself, in your own words, something you have learned. To do retrieval practice, you first read a text and then describe the main ideas in your own words. You can even quiz yourself and ask yourself out loud what questions might come up from this section. If possible, you should also connect the new information with what you have previously learned. Although this method is time-consuming, it is an effective way to learn and memorize new information and also to ensure you understand the text you just read. Using this method in combination with other techniques allows for more cognitive effort, which results in higher levels of conceptual learning and application of the knowledge[8].

Retrieval practice could also be done by writing down or summarizing the content on a piece of paper. Writing things down uses additional parts of your brain, meaning that you're making an effort to consciously reproduce information that you learned before without the help of cues[8].

Remember that actively recalling information does not always have to be successful in the beginning. In fact, it could be extremely difficult to recall content the first couple of times you read it. However, even unsuccessful attempts to bring information from your memory are believed to enhance learning[13]. So, keep trying and continue the effort even though it might not feel as though you are making any progress at times. Eventually, with enough practice, you will.

QUIZZING YOURSELF

Quizzes are common in medical school. Typically, there are questions for you to answer at the end of a section, a full chapter, or an entire book. Answering questions after a section of text accompanied by feedback enhances learning[14]. Quizzes improve not only your memory but also your understanding, as your brain starts to process the information to solve a problem. A quiz will help you to recall information that you have read and also reinforces your memory by forcing you to apply it in a clinical setting. Quizzes are also good to do because the typical questions center around the most important information on a given topic. Therefore, doing quizzes should be a big part of your studies and done regularly. Interestingly, being quizzed about content that you have not read before is also shown to enhance your learning of that content[13–20].

But quizzing yourself does not always have to involve using questions from your textbook, your teacher, or the Internet. After you read a text, write down all the questions that you think could be important for each section. Then write down your answers to them and quiz yourself this way. By doing so, you will focus not only on the most important questions that may be asked on your exam but also on knowledge that you might have difficulty remembering[14–20].

Studies also show that quizzing is superior to passive book learning because an equivalent learning success can be reached in *less than half the time*. Challenging tests and quizzes are thought of as discouraging to students; however, studies demonstrate that although difficult tests produce high error rates at first, they actually *stimulate subsequent learning*[14–20].

TESTING METHOD

The testing method simply means that you recall the information to yourself with a test after you have read a list of words or a text. Even though many studies have found retesting to be more effective than restudying for long-term memory retention, many students seem to be unaware of this or still do not do it as frequently as they should[21].

In one study, a group of students was instructed to study a list of 40 words four times with short breaks in between, while another group studied the list of words only once and then took free recall tests afterwards. The researchers found that the second group of students remembered the words better than the first group did[22].

In another study, researchers carried out a randomized controlled trial involving a didactic conference for pediatric and emergency medicine residents. The study demonstrated that repeated testing resulted in significantly higher long-term retention than repeated studying. Students' final test scores were on average 13% higher in the group that did repeated testing[23].

Therefore, when you study, try to incorporate the testing method by reading a text and then testing yourself frequently. You can do this by writing the questions and answers yourself. But if you want an easier approach, just read a section and then start asking yourself questions in your head to make yourself recall the information.

SPACED REPETITION

We know that repetition is the basis of all knowledge retention. As I mentioned before, the way we perform the repetition also matters[24]. Many studies have shown that spaced repetition is beneficial[24]. A study done on students who were studying immunology and reproductive physiology demonstrated this concept. A group of 250 students was divided into five smaller groups: two of the groups actively recalled the knowledge at a *steady* interval, and two groups actively recalled the information at *expanding* intervals. The fifth group served as a control group. The two groups that recalled the knowledge at expanding intervals had a significantly greater recall of facts on the final test at 29 days, even higher than that of the groups that recalled the concepts with steady intervals, but both groups performed twice as well as the control group[24].

Another study showed similar results. Thirty subjects studied information about Antarctica in either steady or expanded intervals[25]. During the final test after 1 week, the group that studied at expanding intervals outperformed the group that recalled information at a steady interval by a two-to-one margin. Interestingly, in between the intervals, both groups studied information about other regions such as Africa and Greenland. The authors concluded that expanding interval retrieval practice improved students' long-term memory of *correct* information, and in fact helped to prevent the learning of *incorrect* information.

We can draw two major conclusions here that you can also apply to your studying. First, retrieval practice after your first learning session is a core contributor to successful learning, just as was stated earlier regarding active recall and the testing method. Second, doing retrieval practice at expanding intervals seems to significantly enhance learning.

YOUR BREATHING

More often than not during your years in medical school, you will feel stressed when you sit down to study. Time is short, and you are conscious of needing to rapidly learn new information before your exams. Stress has a very real impact on your ability to focus and learn. When you are stressed, your body produces too much noradrenaline—a stress hormone that gets released when we focus, get emotional, or enter other mental states where we need to increase our attention—making it harder for you to focus and negatively affecting your memory retention. This is where your breath comes into play. According to one study, participants who had better synchronization between their attention and their breathing—those who took deep breaths at regular intervals—showed lower levels of noradrenaline, which was believed to enhance their learning. In short, it appears that our attention is influenced by how we breathe. By regulating your breathing, you can optimize your focus and therefore improve your memory[26].

So, when you are studying, focus on your breathing from time to time. Try to take deep breaths at regular intervals (Figure 11.3). This technique improves your focus and synchronizes your breathing. Remembering to notice your breathing could be difficult at first, but just being aware of your breath can make a difference. This is one of the techniques that worked for me.

FOCUS

It goes without saying that you need to focus during your study sessions. Just remember that in order to optimize your learning, you have to be completely focused. And the more focused you are, the better you will learn[4]. Most people focus best in the morning, but this varies from person to person. Find the time of day when you focus best and try to always study at that time. Moreover, as you have been reminded many times in this book, distraction is the enemy of focus. Therefore, remove everything from your study environment that could distract you—your phone, social media, and so on. Most seemingly "urgent" things—texting, emails, messages, and even phone calls—do not require your immediate attention and can therefore easily be dealt with later in the day.

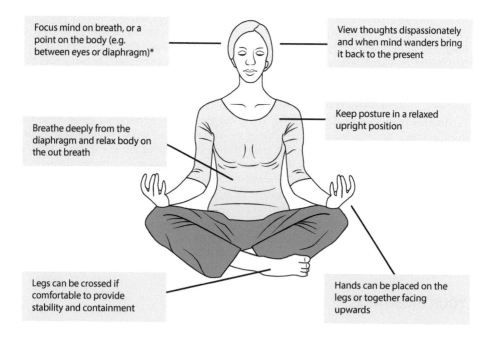

Focus mind on breath, or a point on the body (e.g. between eyes or diaphragm)*

View thoughts dispassionately and when mind wanders bring it back to the present

Breathe deeply from the diaphragm and relax body on the out breath

Keep posture in a relaxed upright position

Legs can be crossed if comfortable to provide stability and containment

Hands can be placed on the legs or together facing upwards

*After 5–15 minutes of 'focused attention', mindfulness awareness can optionally be alternatively extended to external environment (present location and sounds) or 'open monitoring' of internal thoughts (dispassionate observation).

Fig. 11.3 Mindfulness meditation. (Reused with permission from Sarris J, Wardle J. *Clinical Naturopathy: an Evidence-Based Guide to Practice*, 3rd ed. Elsevier; 2019. Figure 14.2.)

If you lose your focus, that's okay. Just be aware that you have lost it and try to refocus. Even if you do have to do this 100 times during a study session, don't get stressed out about it. Everyone loses their focus, but you already know that it can be improved through practice, by refocusing until your attention span lengthens.

COMPREHENSION

Your knowledge retention is best when you attempt to understand the information you read. This point cannot be overstated. Sure, there will be things that will be difficult to understand and just have to be memorized, but most things in medicine have concepts to comprehend. Therefore, your goal should always be to understand something, because once you do, your memory of that information will also be so much better[4,7]. You should first seek to understand the information you are learning, connect the dots, and develop a true understanding of the text you have read and only then try to memorize the details through the methods I have explained here.

ACRONYMS AND MNEMONICS

This is an old and relatively well-known method of memorization. With this technique, the first letter of a word is used to form another word that is easy to remember. This technique can be used for single words or to string together a complete sentence. Box 11.1 presents a well-known mnemonic that medical students often use to learn the 12 cranial nerves.

We can go even further than just learning the names of things. To continue with the example of cranial nerves, we can also learn the function of each nerve. In this case, does the nerve have a motor function, sensory function, or both? This is an effective way to memorize information that is linked together. Every time you want to recall the name or function of the cranial nerves, just recall the mnemonic first; you will eventually be able to name everything on free recall. You can find many popular mnemonics online by searching for "medical mnemonics" or "medical acronyms."

CREATING A FEELING

Emotions play a central role in the formation of memories. This is why people can remember traumatic events in great detail. When we go into fight, flight, fright, or freeze, a part of the brain called the amygdala is activated, the same area that enhances our memory. A study done on

---

BOX 11.1 ■ A Mnemonic Used to Learn the 12 Cranial Nerves

Oh, Oh, Oh, To Touch And Feel, Very Good Vibes, Ah Ha
nervus **o**pticus
nervus **o**lfactorius
nervus **o**culomotorius
nervus **t**rochlearis
nervus **t**rigeminus
nervus **a**bducens
nervus **f**acialis
nervus **v**estibulocochlearis
nervus **g**lossopharyngeus
nervus **v**agus
nervus **a**ccessorius
nervus **h**ypoglossus

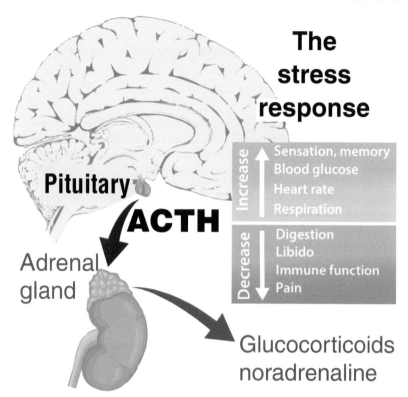

Fig. 11.4 The stress response. (Reused with permission from Garcia-Rill, E. *Arousal in Neurological and Psychiatric Diseases*. Academic Press; 2019. Figure 5.1.)

115 subjects split in two groups found that the group shown images that triggered an emotional reaction remembered the images better than the group shown neutral images[27]. When you feel a strong emotion, you activate the amygdala; that leads to the secretion of adrenaline, a stress hormone that stimulates the hippocampus, the memory center of the brain, thereby enhancing your memory (Figure 11.4).

How can you take advantage of this hormonal cascade to improve your studies? In many cases, it is all about being creative. When you learn about a disease, you can think about a person who has that disease or remember a clinical rotation where you saw a person with that disease. Alternatively, you can pinch your arm or yell a word out loud when you are memorizing information, and the emotions elicited by those actions may help to make that memory stick.

INTERLEAVING

Many students study by reading about one topic and then jumping to the next topic. This approach isn't wrong. In fact, it might be the only way you *can* study certain material. The technique of interleaving, however, involves frequently switching between topics on purpose. For example, if you are studying both pharmacology and histology for an exam, you would switch from one topic to the other instead of first reading all the content on pharmacology and then all the content on histology. This technique forces your brain to make connections between the topics, including any overlapping knowledge, and helps to cement the information in your brain[28,29].

SUMMARY OF TECHNIQUES

You now have a whole arsenal of memorization and learning techniques at your disposal. It might seem overwhelming if you assume that you have to incorporate every technique every time you study. But this is not the case. The key is to try each of the techniques to see which ones work best for you and for which purposes. Play with them and mix them up as you go. With experimentation, you will discover which ones serve you best. Remember that many of the techniques can be used simultaneously and that the more effort you put into trying different methods, the better your chances of quickly retaining the information.

Summary

- A good memory is essential for learning the enormous volume of information presented to you in medical school. However, your memory, like many other things, can be improved through strategic practice.
- You already have a decent memory to begin with, as it is part of why you have made it this far. Do not doubt your ability.
- Your belief system—thinking and believing that you have a good memory—helps to improve your ability to memorize.
- Repetition is the foundation to memorizing information, but the way in which you do your rounds of repetition makes a big difference.
- Aside from repetition, other techniques shown to improve your memory are understanding the information, association, chunking, visualization, flashcards, retrieval practice, quizzing yourself, testing, spaced repetition, your breathing, focus, comprehension, acronyms and mnemonics, creating a feeling, and interleaving.

References

1. Rovers SFE, Stalmeijer RE, van Merriënboer JJG, Savelberg HHCM, de Bruin ABH. How and why do students use learning strategies? A mixed methods study on learning strategies and desirable difficulties with effective strategy users. *Front Psychol.* 2018;9:2501. https://doi.org/10.3389/fpsyg.2018.02501.
2. Shirani Bidabadi N, Nasr Isfahani A, Rouhollahi A, Khalili R. Effective teaching methods in higher education: requirements and barriers. *J Adv Med Educ Prof.* 2016;4(4):170–178.
3. Corell A, Regueras LM, Verdú E, Verdú MJ, de Castro JP. Effects of competitive learning tools on medical students: a case study. *PLoS One.* 2018;13(3). https://doi.org/10.1371/journal.pone.0194096.
4. Bisaz R, Travaglia A, Alberini CM. The neurobiological bases of memory formation: from physiological conditions to psychopathology. *Psychopathology.* 2014;47(6):347–356. https://doi.org/10.1159/000363702.
5. Schmidmaier R, Eiber S, Ebersbach R, et al. Learning the facts in medical school is not enough: which factors predict successful application of procedural knowledge in a laboratory setting? *BMC Med Educ.* 2013;13:28. https://doi.org/10.1186/1472-6920-13-28.
6. Radcliffe C, Lester H. Perceived stress during undergraduate medical training: a qualitative study. *Med Educ.* 2003;37(1):32–38.
7. Friedlander MJ, Andrews L, Armstrong EG, et al. What can medical education learn from the neurobiology of learning? *Acad Med.* 2011;86(4):415–420.
8. Augustin M. How to learn effectively in medical school: test yourself, learn actively, and repeat in intervals. *Yale J Biol Med.* 2014;87(2):207–212.
9. Ebbinghaus H. Ueber das Gedaechtnis: Untersuchungen zur experimentellen Psychologie. [About memory: a contribution to experimental psychology]. Duncker & Humblot; 1885. German.
10. Ericsson KA, Chase WG, Faloon S. Acquisition of a memory skill. *Science.* 1980;208(4448):1181–1182.
11. Fowler A, Whitehurst K, Al Omran Y, et al. How to study effectively. *Int J Surg Oncol (NY).* 2017;2(6):e31. https://doi.org/10.1097/IJ9.0000000000000031.
12. Solopchuk O, Alamia A, Olivier E, Zénon A. Chunking improves symbolic sequence processing and relies on working memory gating mechanisms. *Learn Mem.* 2016;23(3):108–112.

13. Kornell N, Hays MJ, Bjork RA. Unsuccessful retrieval attempts enhance subsequent learning. *J Exp Psychol Learn Mem Cogn.* 2009;35(4):989–998.
14. Azorlosa JW. (2011). The effect of announced quizzes on exam performance: II. *J Instr Psychol.* 2011;38:3–7.
15. Batsell WR Jr, Perry JL, Hanley E, Hostetter AB. Ecological validity of the testing effect: the use of daily quizzes in introductory psychology. *Teach Psychol.* 2016;44(1):18–23. https://doi.org/10.1177/0098628316677492.
16. Braun KW, Sellers RD. Using a "daily motivational quiz" to increase student preparation, attendance and participation. *Issues Account Educ.* 2012;27(1):267–279.
17. Hardsell L. The effect of quiz timing on exam performance. *J Educ Bus.* 2009;84(3):135–141.
18. Hatteberg SJ, Steffy K. Increasing reading compliance of undergraduates: an evaluation of compliance methods. *Teach Sociol.* 2013;41(4):346–352.
19. Johnson BC, Kiviniemi MT. The effect of online chapter quizzes on exam performance in an undergraduate social psychology course. *Teach Psychol.* 2009;36(1):33–37.
20. Kouyoumdjian H. Influence of unannounced quizzes and cumulative final on attendance and study behavior. *Teach Psychol.* 2004;31(2):110–111.
21. Schmidmaier R, Ebersbach R, Schiller M, Hege I, Holzer M, Fischer MR. Using electronic flashcards to promote learning in medical students: retesting versus restudying. *Med Educ.* 2011;45(11):1101–1110.
22. Hogan RM, Kintsch W. Differential effects of study and test trials on long-term recognition and recall. *J Verbal Learning Verbal Behav.* 1971;10:562–567.
23. Larsen DP, Butler AC, Roediger HL III. Repeated testing improves long-term retention relative to repeated study: a randomized controlled trial. *Med Educ.* 2009;43(12):1174–1181.
24. Dobson JL. Effect of uniform versus expanding retrieval practice on the recall of physiology information. *Adv Physiol Educ.* 2012;36(1):6–12.
25. Storm BC, Bjork RA, Storm JC. Optimizing retrieval as a learning event: when and why expanding retrieval practice enhances long-term retention. *Mem Cognit.* 2010;38(2):244–253.
26. Melnychuk MC, Dockree PM, O'Connell RG, Murphy PR, Balsters JH, Robertson IH. Coupling of respiration and attention via the locus coeruleus: effects of meditation and pranayama. *Psychophysiology.* 2018;55(9):e13091. https://doi.org/10.1111/psyp.13091.
27. Tambini A, Rimmele U, Phelps EA, Davachi L. Emotional brain states carry over and enhance future memory formation. *Nat Neurosci.* 2017;20(2):271–278.
28. Rohrer D. Interleaving helps students distinguish among similar concepts. *Educ Psychol Rev.* 2012;24:355–367.
29. Rohrer D, Taylor K. The shuffling of mathematics problems improves learning. *Instr Sci.* 2007;35:481–498.

CHAPTER 12

Strategies for Medical School Examinations

By failing to prepare, you are preparing to fail.
—Benjamin Franklin

Hope for the best, prepare for the worst
—Chris Bradford

CHAPTER OUTLINE

Introduction

Exam anxiety is something all students experience in medical school. You will feel a lot of pressure before, during, and after exams owing to the great importance placed on your grades. It's natural to feel anxious—exams *are* important. Your grades can have significant consequences for your future, especially how well you do on the USMLE (United States Medical Licensing Examination). If you get a failing grade, then you may not match into a residency training program. If you get a lower than average score, you may have difficulties matching. There is a lot at stake. If you have a great score, you will most likely have a much better interview and matching outcome.

Doing well on your exams is one thing. Being a good test-taker is quite another. Doing well on an exam requires intensive practice and preparation. Similarly, being a good test-taker is not just a matter of possessing raw talent. It has a lot to do with employing the right strategies and tactics: how you study, how you mentally prepare, how you take your exam, and so on. This chapter will help you learn the best test-taking strategies so that you can ace your exams.

Exams in medical school are different from those in other programs. You will have the familiar paper-based exams, where you need to answer questions; you will have multiple choice questions; and you will have clinical exams with patient encounters; and you will have written and oral reports[1]. Each type of test is important to master and requires a different strategy. If you go into these tests blindly, without any preparation, then your performance and thus your grades will likely suffer[1].

Exam Preparation

Your best bet when it comes to performing well on a test is preparation[2,3]. It may sound obvious, but lack of preparation is the main reason why things do not go well. To score high on a test, you must gain solid knowledge of a subject by studying everything necessary before test day. If you do that and are also well prepared, there will typically be no or very few unpleasant surprises. If you do not prepare well, then you are in for a bumpy ride[2-5].

If you take medical school seriously, then you have no excuse as to why you are not prepared before an exam. You should always create a study plan and follow it, beginning far in advance to make sure you don't run out of time. Top athletes know that winning doesn't start by performing well the day of the actual competition; winning starts months or years earlier, with the hard work and constant training that set you up to eventually win. The same goes for exams success in medical school—it is your careful advance preparations that will give you the high scores you're aiming for[2-5].

Find Out Exactly What's Covered on the Exam

In order to get a high score on your exam, you have to know what content will be covered. It can be difficult to know what it will be with 100% certainty, yet plenty of students still manage to achieve high scores because they are strategic in their preparation. So, to the best of your knowledge, find out everything you are expected to know. What specific topics are more important than others? What questions are typically repeated? Do some digging: Read the information sheets, check with classmates and teachers on possible exam content, and don't be satisfied with the information until it's crystal clear to you.

And if you feel unsure, ask again. Mention to your teacher that you are aiming to do well, and ask whether there are any specific chapters, areas, or knowledge that you should focus on more to get a better score. Don't be ashamed to ask. You have the right to ask for and receive this information.

Once you are equipped with the right information, you will know which areas to focus on when you sit down to study. That doesn't mean you shouldn't learn the other content equally well, but at least you'll know what to concentrate on[4,5]. This strategy will make the actual task of studying that much easier, especially if you follow my study methods.

Tactics Before Your Exams

SOLVE PROBLEMS AND ANSWER QUESTIONS

Most courses have a question bank that teachers can pick questions from in order to create exams. While some teachers choose to come up with their own questions, they still compare the level of difficulty and question content with those from the question banks or on previous exams. Thus, their questions will usually be inspired by old exams or information from your textbook.

Learning is not simply a matter of reading and memorizing the information contained within the pages of a textbook. While reading and memorization are important, you also need to structure and process the knowledge so that you can analyze it logically. One way of doing that is to answer questions. This is an ingenious way of learning that helps the knowledge stick in your brain[6]. Answering questions and solving problems also makes it easier for you to connect your new learning with previous knowledge so that you develop a broader as well as deeper understanding of an area. Another advantage of answering questions and solving problems is that it gives you a feel for what you do not know. Your inability to answer certain questions or problems should motivate you to return to the textbook in order to review that information more precisely. If you do enough questions, problems, and previous test questions/exams, you will end up reviewing most of the knowledge that will be covered on your upcoming exam. Studies show that answering questions from question banks leads students to score higher on their exams[6].

I always practiced old test questions, which meant that I usually recognized most of the questions on the actual exam pretty quickly. At times, I remember seeing questions that were identical to those that appeared on previous tests, which essentially gave me "free" points.

SKIM THROUGH THE TEXTBOOK

One way to ensure that you know the content inside out before your test or exam is to skim through all the relevant pages of your textbook or lecture notes. As you skim the pages, make sure that you know all the content; if not, then read and reread that part to learn it. A few days before your test, you should have a solid foundation. The last few days before the test, you typically don't have time to reread all the pages again. And most of the time, you won't need to. If you have been following your study plan, then you likely already know most of it, but there are often a few details that you still need to clarify. So, focus on the areas that are not yet embedded in your brain and try to learn them. This will also give you a quick repetition of the knowledge that you already know[4,5].

GET ENOUGH SLEEP THE DAY BEFORE

You should not be tired or sleep deprived when writing an exam. Your focus and concentration should be at their best, so get the best sleep you can the night before. Fatigue and sleepiness will affect your focus negatively as well as your attention to detail. Sleep is something that many students usually skimp on during their medical school years. Even if you must do it at times, do your best not to the night before an exam. Make sure you get at least 6 hours of sleep, and preferably longer, so that you feel alert and refreshed when you wake up the day of your test.

Staying up all night to cram before the day of the test is not something I recommend. You will be so tired that all those extra hours learning will not have been anywhere close to effective. At that point, three cups of coffee won't help you any better. In fact, coffee might actually make you more anxious rather than more focused. To not sleep at all the night before your exam is taking a huge risk that will likely backfire. Your focus, concentration, and memory will all suffer. I advise against all-night studying as a preparation strategy. You should know the content of your textbook or notes well in advance of the exam. Therefore, you shouldn't need to stay up all night just to squeeze in a few extra hours of studying.

One thing you can do, however, is to sleep around 6 hours and then get up a few hours earlier in the morning to look through your notes and textbooks one last time before the test to memorize the small details.

BUILD MENTAL FOCUS

On the day of the exam, make sure you wake up early, eat a healthy breakfast, and come to the exam room well in advance. The last thing you want is unnecessary stress the day of your exam.

Mild to moderate stress can be beneficial for your focus, but high levels of stress hormones, as I have already explained, will negatively affect your attention and memory and can cause you to miss important details on your test[5,7,8]. Therefore, don't give yourself anything extra to worry about by waking up late, missing the bus, or not arriving on time because of bad weather.

Bring a pen, a pencil, and an eraser; turn off your phone; and find a place to sit. Be calm and present. A little nervousness is okay, as it means your brain is alert and ready to face the challenge of the exam, but try to manage your nervousness by keeping your breath slow and steady.

Once you sit down to do your test, do not let your mind wander. Forget about what you are doing tomorrow, the fight you had with a friend, or what's going on this coming weekend. Moreover, don't think about borrowing a pen or that you might have put too little money in the parking meter. Get into the zone: focus fully on the subject you're about to be tested on and think about how you will answer the questions that come up[5,7,8].

I will never forget the way one of my classmates acted the morning of an exam. I noticed that his body language was extremely still. During every break, he would sit in his chair and stare at the wall. When it was time to reenter the exam room after a break, he would calmly rise and walk back to his seat with his head held high. I asked him, "Has anything happened?" He looked me straight in the eyes and replied, "No, Raman. I'm just very focused." He got an A on that test.

My friend's demeanor inspired me. He made me understand that body language and behavior are connected to focus, which then correlates with performance on an exam. If you joke around too much and chitchat with everyone around you, you may very well lose that feeling of "being in the zone." So, do not flutter about and distract yourself right before the test or during a break, expecting that a few minutes later you will resume being calm, focused, and attentive enough to perform well. Creating maximum focus before an exam takes time. If you start to get worked up before or during this period, your body has to start all over again. Do not waste those precious minutes before your exam. Focus is about much more than sitting quietly in the exam room when you arrive. If you want to maximize your performance on the exam, then you must be prepared to maintain your focus from start to finish[9].

MAINTAIN YOUR ENERGY

In Chapter 14, I discuss the importance of diet and share the potential benefits of fasting in the morning. However, on an exam day, I suggest that you eat a healthy breakfast to give your brain adequate fuel and to ensure that you don't get hungry during your exam. Once your brain signals to you that you are hungry, both your focus and attention can be affected. If you don't eat enough before your exam, then you will have fewer resources remaining for memory and focus. However, you also don't want to eat too much. When you eat a heavy meal, more of your circulation is diverted to your digestive system, a process that may make you feel tired and sleepy. Therefore, eat a moderate-sized meal before the exam.

To maintain your energy during the exam, bring a small piece of chocolate or other sweets that you can snack on every 15 to 30 minutes (if allowed). This way, you can "boost" your blood sugar and energy and thus possibly perform better. But keep in mind that quick-release carbohydrates (such as those found in chocolate) can cause blood sugar to quickly drop, so it's important that you "maintain" a steady blood sugar during the hour(s) that you are writing the test[10,11]. You might also consider bringing a coffee or a mild energy drink to drink 20 to 30 minutes before the exam and to continue sipping during the exam. This will further boost your focus and energy.

Several studies have also shown that concentration, performance, and memory capacity increase when you chew gum. Chewing increases blood circulation in the brain, heart rate, and oxygen uptake by and transport to the brain. It could also help to fight sleepiness[12]. But chew your gum quietly so that you don't disturb others!

BE CALM

As I mentioned earlier, exam anxiety is completely normal and extremely common[4,9]. However, if your anxiety is too high, it may negatively affect your focus. Your body's stress hormones can increase to levels that adversely affect your attention and memory. When you feel too much anxiety, you may get so amped up that you label that "nervous" feeling in your body as something bad, which in turn could result in your having thoughts about failing the exam or performing badly. You then begin to worry about worrying. This cycle continues and sometimes results in panic attacks.

Before going any further, it's essential that you understand the body's natural response to stress. Stress is a normal cortical reaction in your brain that occurs in response to a real or perceived threat; your brain cannot actually tell the difference. Since there is no real threat in your case—you are mainly keyed up because of the exam—you are in no danger if your heart rate goes up, you start breathing faster, you get anxious, or you experience other symptoms[4,9]. Do not panic! Stress is simply your body's way of preparing you for an important event: your exam. You should be feeling a little bit of nervousness, or the "good" kind of stress. Moreover, if you breathe slowly and deeply, your anxiety will soon dissipate.

Here are the best ways to manage exam anxiety:

1. Practice and prepare before your exam. If you have practiced, then you have nothing to worry about. Remind yourself of this fact.
2. Do not let yourself get caught up in a loop of catastrophic thoughts. The worst thing that can happen is that you don't perform as well as you wanted to. Sure, it's not ideal and you will feel disappointed, but there are often ways to make up for this later. Regardless, it won't help if you plunge yourself into a black hole by thinking the worst.
3. Breathe slowly and deeply. Do this both before and during the exam. As soon as you get anxious, close your eyes for a few moments and just focus on your breathing.
4. Think happy thoughts. Positive thinking will definitely move you into a better mental space. Think about something that automatically makes you smile or feel at peace and focus on those thoughts or images.

Tactics During Your Exam

ONE QUESTION AT A TIME

After you sit down to write your exam, close your eyes and take a deep breath before looking at the first question. Some students like to look at all the questions on the exam before they start to answer the first question. This is fine if it is something you are accustomed to doing, but this could also create unnecessary stress and confusion for you. You may read a question you feel unsure about, which will make you feel worried and scared. In addition, you can lose time by getting stuck on a question as you reflect on whether or not you know the answer. It is therefore usually best to start from the beginning and answer one question at a time[13,14].

READ EACH QUESTION AT LEAST TWICE

Read the first question at least twice before beginning to answer it. You should do this partly to make sure that you have both understood the question correctly and not misunderstood any of the details. Sometimes, it is the smallest details that can make the difference between the right and wrong answer. You also decrease the risk of having to erase and rewrite or second-guess your answers, which can save you a lot of time. A common mistake students make is to misunderstand the question, leading them to answer a different question from the one that was being asked. You will lose many points for doing this. Therefore, read the questions carefully and many times if needed. Furthermore, if possible, ask your teacher to explain the question if you do not understand it[13,14].

If you are stumped about a question, stop and read it slowly several times. When you read a question repeatedly, it can prompt your brain to recall related knowledge. Review your memories of each page you have read and try to remember what the details were. Consider whether any of the content that you read might have something to do with the question. If you use these methods systematically, then you will usually come up with something to write or an answer to choose for the question[13,14]. The key is avoid getting panicked and worried that you don't immediately know the answer. Some exam questions are meant to be more challenging than others, and that's okay. If all the questions were easy and everyone could easily answer them, then what would be the point of exams?

In the worst-case scenario, if you really do not know the answer to the question, then make an educated guess. Never leave a question blank. Even if you earn only half a point, it's better than nothing. And if you do not get it right, at least you know you tried. Therefore, write anything related to the topic. Personally, when I didn't know the answer to a question, I used to always write a summary of everything that I knew about the topic. In 99% of cases, I always got at least half a point!

REVIEW YOUR ANSWERS

Once you have written your answer, read through the question again and make sure that you have responded to everything correctly. The more details you write down and the better your reasoning—especially when you're not 100% sure of the answer—the greater the chances are that you will earn more points and a higher grade at the end. Of course, sometimes you may not have the complete answer to the question, but if you write down as much as you can about what you do know, then you are much more likely to get that part of the answer right. If it is a multiple choice question, you can simply reread the question to make sure you have understood the background before you answer[13,14].

After you have finished reading all the questions and answers and feel as though you're done with the exam—Wait! Your first instinct will be to just submit it and exit the exam hall. You are drained and eager to get it over with. But take it easy. Make one last effort: go through the entire test once more. Never leave the examination room early. It's a good thing if you have a lot of time remaining because it gives you the opportunity to double-check all your answers. Start by reading each question from the beginning and then reading all your answers. Read your answers critically, correct any errors you discover, and make sure your answers are easy to read for the teacher. The last thing you want is for your teacher to misunderstand you because of how you have phrased things. If it is a multiple choice question exam, make sure you read the questions again quickly and review your answers. If you feel that you have a better guess on a question you are unsure about, then pick that answer. Trust that it is worth the extra time you spend at the end, however exhausted you may be. This will be the last chance you get to review this exam… forever. Think about that. I cannot recall a single exam in medical school where I did not correct at least one of my answers during this final review. I went through every single exam I had in the end and always found things that I could edit. You likely will too.

Strategies for Different Types of Questions and Exams

FACTUAL QUESTIONS

Never write personal opinions if you are asked a factual question. Write down the facts in as detailed a way as possible. The more you can demonstrate that you can provide the requested information, the smarter—and more knowledgeable—you will appear.

ESSAY QUESTIONS

Here you should mix facts with your own opinions. Essay questions require you to show that you can discuss, reason, and draw conclusions. Discuss advantages and disadvantages. Argue for and against. Describe consequences, similarities, and differences. That's what will earn you the higher grade. Use your imagination and be creative. But remember, your points must be relevant to the question. You don't discuss the mating rituals of elephants in Southern Africa when you have an essay question on pharmacology—unless you can make an extremely good connection. This may sound like an absurd example, but I know students who have made far more irrelevant connections and conclusions than that. You should be perceived as knowledgeable and professional, and your discussions should elevate you as a person and show your intelligence.

DETAILED QUESTIONS

When answering detailed questions, dig into your memory to retrieve all the knowledge you possess on a given topic. Read the chapter on memorization and learning techniques as well as the study techniques section of this book and you should have a good handle on how to approach this type of question. If you can't answer a detailed question, you should make approximations—that is, an approximate estimate of the answer. Anatomy is an example of a course with a lot of detailed knowledge that can be challenging to learn. You may be asked questions related to structures that you've never heard of or even forgot about. But there are often ways to estimate the answer. For instance, if you know that the bones of the forearm are called the radius and ulna, then it is reasonable for you to assume that the corresponding nerves are called the radial and ulnar nerves. It is always better to make a qualified estimate, guess, or approximation than not to answer at all.

MULTIPLE CHOICE QUESTIONS—MMQ TEST

Multiple choice questions, or MMQ tests and exams, are common in medical school and being used with increasing frequency. MMQ essentially means that you are asked a question and offered some options to choose from for the correct answer. There are a couple of ways to approach this type of question[2,15]. You can read the question and then the answers *or* you can read all the answers first and then read the question.

My strategy has always been to read the answer choices first before I read the question. I read the answers first for a couple of reasons:

- Many times, the questions can be long, and some of the information that the teacher includes might actually be irrelevant. By reading the answers first, you can quickly sort out which information is relevant.
- By reading the answers first, you may understand the question better as well as the context while your brain has already verified the answer choices. Thus, you may be able to answer a question more quickly. This approach allows you to automatically establish connections. As you switch from reading the answers to reading the question, your brain matches the question with an answer and "looks" for other clues to further back up your chosen answer.

Here are other things to keep in mind about MMQ tests:

- Immediately eliminate answer options that you know are incorrect with 100% certainty so that you have as few answers as possible to choose from.
- Do not change your answer once you have chosen it, unless you are absolutely sure that your change is correct. Your answers are more likely to be correct the first time. However, if you decide that you made a mistake when you go back to review your answers, then you should definitely change it.

- You have a limited time to answer each question and you must be fairly quick about it, so try to follow this systematic approach:
  - Read the answers.
  - Read the question.
  - Eliminate all incorrect answers.
  - Choose the answer you think is right.
  - Put a checkmark next to a question if you are unsure and return to it later.
  - Move on to the next question.
  - When you have completed all the questions, go back to the questions you were unsure of and double-check your answers.

You should practice keeping the whole process of answering a question to less than 1.5 minutes per question. Do not spend too long on any one question. Either you know the answer or you don't. Sometimes, when we are under pressure, it can take some time to retrieve the correct information. Instead of getting stuck on one question for too long, put a checkmark next to that question and come back to it later.

ORAL EXAMS

You should study just as hard for an oral exam as a written one. Try to predict the questions that will be asked and practice in advance how you would respond to each question. As part of your exam preparation, write down your answers in point form to guide you in the right direction when you eventually do your oral exam. These could include what you are going to say for each question and also how to answer in a well-rounded and articulate manner. Practice your entire response in front of a mirror several times. You can even ask someone to listen to you and offer you constructive feedback to improve your delivery[5].

Knowing the format of the exam is also important. You will want to know how the exam is structured; whether there are numbered bays relating to distinct anatomical areas or body systems; how many bays there will be; how long you will have in each bay; and how that time is divided into examination, presentation, and questions[5].

On the day of your oral exam, always arrive on time, be dressed appropriately, turn off your phone, and be polite by saying "Hello," "How are you?," and "Thank you" before, during, and after the oral exam. Address your evaluator as "Dr.". Everyone likes a well-mannered person. Make sure you maintain good posture and be confident but humble. Shake hands with your evaluator and introduce yourself. You do not want to come across as overconfident or cocky[5].

Before responding to a question from your examiner, pause for a few seconds. Try to understand the question well. Many times, students provide an answer that is unrelated to the question being asked because they did not listen carefully enough. If you do this, you may be perceived as having difficulty understanding or not being sharp enough. You do not want to give that impression. If you didn't hear something or were unclear about what was being asked, then ask the examiner to repeat the question. Then quickly assess how you are going to answer the question in a structured and organized format.

Look for clues. If there is a glass of water near the patient, think thyroid; if there is a sheet of paper, think nerve injury and test for muscle power. Do not, however, rely too much on clues, since the items may have been left there by a patient from the morning session or are there to mislead you[5].

Remember that oral exams are also about your social skills. Many times, it is more important *how* you respond to something rather than making sure that you provide all the details. Always look your teacher in the eye and respond with confidence. Importantly, avoid the following:

- Using words like "uh" or "um"
- Being nervous

- Responding with incomplete sentences
- Looking down or away
- Being impolite
- Coming across as distant or with stiff body language
- Speaking in a dull or monotonous tone of voice

Instead, try to embody the following qualities:

- Charisma
- Warmth
- Enthusiasm
- Confidence
- Politeness

Speak with emphasis so that your words come alive. Try to stand tall and with confident body language, and don't be afraid to gesture with your hands (but don't wave your hands around nervously or wildly).

Time Management

During exams, time management is key. Many students lack good time management skills, which ends up hurting them because they cannot answer all the questions in the time allotted. You risk losing a lot of easy points when you miss out on answering easy questions. Poor time management also creates more stress for you, which can further hurt your score. Managing your time during an exam is essential and, quite frankly, pretty easy. I will share a few simple steps on how to do it[16].

First, determine how many minutes the exam is. Second, review how many questions your exam contains. Third, calculate how long you can spend on each question. Always try to leave at least 10 minutes in the end to read through your answers.

Here's an example:

- Time for test: 60 minutes
- Number of questions: 50
- Reserved time for review: 10 minutes
- Total allocated time: 60 − 10 = 50 minutes
- Time per question: 50 questions / 50 minutes = 1 minute per question + 10 minutes reserved time for final review

This is an extremely easy way to figure out how long you can spend on each question before you start your exam. Ideally, you should get this information before the exam so that you are prepared. However, the instructions on the length of the exam and the number of questions may only be revealed when the exam starts. Once you have done your calculation, start answering the questions and keep an eye on the clock so that you stay within the allotted time frame for each question. Keep in mind that some questions will require more time from you and some will require less time. If you stick to about 1 minute per question, then it will work out in the end. However, if you know that you don't have more than 1 minute per question, you should really not spend more than twice or at most three times more than that on a question. If you do find yourself spending a long time on a question, you should add a checkmark next to the question to review it later and move on. This way, you can be sure that you will be able to handle all the questions without stress. In addition, you will ensure that you leave nothing blank.

If, despite your time management efforts, you discover that you are still running out of time and have a few unanswered questions, follow my prioritizing tips:

- Quickly review all the unanswered questions.
- Check off the questions that are easiest to answer and do them first.
- Move on to the rest of the questions and try to answer them as quickly as you can.

Certain exams are not computerized, so when the time is up, you can try to squeeze a few more minutes into finishing your review of your exam while waiting for the teacher to collect the papers from all the students in the exam room. Ideally, if you have prepared well and managed your time, you should be able to finish with time to spare. However, if you find yourself in a jam, then you can take advantage of those extra few minutes to answer questions while the teacher collects everyone's exam.

Summary

- Make sure you are prepared for your exam. Study and prepare properly and use appropriate study technique from Section II of this book.
- Find out exactly what will be covered on the exam so that you know exactly what to study.
- Do many practice tests using old exams and answer relevant questions. It will help you to process the knowledge you already have. Also, you usually get to answer questions that will appear on your upcoming exam, so you will know some answers in advance.
- Be sure to sleep well the night before the test and do not arrive late.
- Eat just before the test so you do not get hungry during the test. Always have a piece of chocolate with you and a coffee or energy drink to "boost" your energy intermittently.
- Mental and physical focus is important and takes a while to build up right before an exam. Therefore, make sure you maintain your focus and concentration both before and during the exam.
- During the exam itself, read each question twice, try to understand the question, and only then answer. Read through the question and your answer again to check that you have answered the entire question.
- Never leave a question blank. It is always better to write something or take an educated guess than leave a question blank.
- When you have completed the exam, read all your answers again before submitting your paper.
- Know what strategies to use for different types of questions and exams.
- Develop good time management skills to maximize your exam performance. Before you start doing your exam, make sure you know how much time you can allot to each question.

References

1. Howard A. *Types of Medical School Exams. Kaplan.* https://www.kaptest.com/study/usmle/types-of-medical-school-exams/. Accessed 29 September 2020.
2. Walsh K. How to pass exams: evidence-based advice? *J R Soc Med.* 2005;98(6):294. https://doi.org/10.1258/jrsm.98.6.294.
3. Eckerlein N, Roth A, Engelschalk T, Steuer G, Schmitz B, Dresel M. The role of motivational regulation in exam preparation: results from a standardized diary study. *Front Psychol.* 2019;10:81. https://doi.org/10.3389/fpsyg.2019.00081.
4. Yusefzadeh H, Amirzadeh Iranagh J, Nabilou B. The effect of study preparation on test anxiety and performance: a quasi-experimental study. *Adv Med Educ Pract.* 2019;10:245–251. https://doi.org/10.2147/AMEP.S192053.
5. Cascarini L, Irani M. Surviving a clinical exam: a guide for candidates. *J R Soc Med.* 2005;98(4):174–177. https://doi.org/10.1258/jrsm.98.4.174.
6. Bonasso P, Lucke-Wold B III, Reed Z, Bozek J, Cottrell S. Investigating the impact of preparation strategies on USMLE Step 1 performance. *MedEdPublish.* 2015;4(1):5. https://doi.org/10.15694/mep.2015.004.0005.
7. McManus IC, Richards P, Winder BC, Sproston KA. Clinical experience, performance in final examinations, and learning style in medical students: prospective study. *BMJ.* 1998;316:345–350. https://doi.org/10.1136/bmj.316.7128.345.

8. Wright N, Tanner MS. Medical students' compliance with simple administrative tasks and success in final examinations: retrospective cohort study. *BMJ.* 2002;324:1554–1555. https://doi.org/10.1136/bmj.324.7353.1554.
9. Cho H, Ryu S, Noh J, Lee J. The effectiveness of daily mindful breathing practices on test anxiety of students. *PLoS One.* 2016;11(10). https://doi.org/10.1371/journal.pone.0164822.
10. Kim SY, Sim S, Park B, Kong IG, Kim JH, Choi HG. Dietary habits are associated with school performance in adolescents. *Medicine (Baltimore).* 2016;95(12):e3096. https://doi.org/10.1097/MD.0000000000003096.
11. Barker ME, Blain RJ, Russell JM. The influence of academic examinations on energy and nutrient intake in male university students. *Nutr J.* 2015;14:98. https://doi.org/10.1186/s12937-015-0088-y.
12. Allen AP, Smith AP. Chewing gum: cognitive performance, mood, well-being, and associated physiology. *Biomed Res Int.* 2015;2015. https://doi.org/10.1155/2015/654806.
13. Wong L. *Essential Study Skills.* 4th ed. Houghton Mifflin: Harcourt; 2003. https://college.cengage.com/collegesurvival/wong/essential_study/4e/students/interact_practice.html. Accessed September 28, 2020.
14. West C, Kurz T, Smith S, Graham L. Are study strategies related to medical licensing exam performance? *Int J Med Educ.* 2014;5:199–204. https://doi.org/10.5116/ijme.5439.6491.
15. Gloe D. Study habits and test-taking tips. *Dermatol Nurs.* 1999;11(6):439–449.
16. West C, Sadoski M. Do study strategies predict academic performance in medical school? *Med Educ.* 2011;45(7):696–703. https://doi.org/10.1111/j.1365-2923.2011.03929.x.

CHAPTER 13

Never Give Up

Winners never quit, and quitters never win.
—Vince Lombardi

You just can't beat the person who won't give up.
—Babe Ruth

Introduction

Overnight success is a myth. Whichever actor, athlete, or business mogul you hold up as a paragon of success got to where they are today only after years of struggle and hard work. When people see a break-out star in the film industry, for instance, they are largely unaware that this "overnight success" has nearly always spent an entire decade auditioning and being rejected, attending acting classes at night, and doing whatever it took to pay the bills, including serving grumpy restaurant customers. Overnight success really should be renamed "success 10 years in the making."

One day, when you "make it," people are going to ask you *when* you did it. Your answer should be that while others were partying, playing video games, barhopping, drinking, and sleeping in, you were working hard, studying, making the right decisions, and never giving up. And while people may laugh at you, talk behind your back, or not believe in you, you will learn to deflect all that negative energy and mentally and physically prepare yourself for your future and your ultimate success. The important question is not *when* will you make it but *how* will you make it? You will make it by focusing on your goals and never giving up while other people are busy doing things that will not add value to their lives.

The truth is, if you want to "look good" in front of millions, you have to outdo millions in front of nobody. Achieving success is hard. It's most definitely not easy to perform well day after day after day. It requires a lot of determination, focus, hard work, and the ability to never give up. Why? Because achieving an ambitious and difficult goal is, well, difficult. So if you do not consistently maintain the attitude that you will never give up, then your brain will push you to give up and spend your time on easier things. That's just the way the brain tends to work. You must learn to resist this tendency. I will teach you how to do that next.

Two Salespeople

Think about the last time you encountered a salesperson, either in a store or on the phone. If you observe salespeople, then you will notice that there are two main types. The most common type is the one who gives you a phone call or approaches you and tries to sell you a product or service. Typically, they're trying to sell you something they think can bring you great value. They start by exemplifying the problem and the need or gap in the market. They then pitch you on why you should purchase it. As the customer, you can decide whether you want to buy it or not. If you say no, then they will thank you for your time and walk away (or hang up the phone). The second type of salesperson is the one that does not take no for an answer. They will keep giving you persuasive reasons why you should purchase their product or service and will easily counter all your stated reasons for not wanting to buy it.

Imagine that you and a friend are walking through the city on a beautiful, warm, sunny day and you have some change in your pocket. The small change you have in your pocket has no major bearing on your finances, but of course you would prefer to keep it. Suddenly, a salesperson approaches you on the street. What is the first thought that arises, right there and then? Perhaps you think to yourself, "I don't need anything right now and I don't want to buy anything right now. I'll keep this change and buy myself a soda or an ice cream later on so I can cool down on this warm, sunny day." You say no, you and the salesperson part ways, and you are done with the situation.

But hold on! Imagine the same situation, but now the salesperson comes up to you and says, "Excuse me, I can show you a clear example of how this product will change your life, how much you will benefit from it, and it won't affect your finances that much." In this situation, you might still say, "No thanks." But if the same salesperson continues by saying, "I promise you, just try it! I can show you many others who have tried it and how useful it's been for them. In fact, I will give you a discount if you buy it now and throw another one in for free for your friend." If the product is good and cheap, the number of people who would say "no" this time would likely decrease significantly. In fact, many of us would buy the thing and be done with it. Do you notice the difference?

On the one hand, you have a person who is determined. He will persistently keep pushing you to buy a product or service that he really believes will benefit you once you purchase it. He does not accept no for an answer. He does not give up. On the other hand, you have someone that is passively standing and waiting for things to happen or perhaps asks only once whether you'd like to purchase the product or not and then gives up. The point of this example was to illustrate that, just like the salesperson who successfully closes the deal, success will not merely come to *you*. You have to go to *it*. Success in school takes time, and you will certainly encounter many setbacks and challenges. Things will not always go the way you want or planned. You must accept this as a fact of life and keep fighting through it regardless of how often you fail a test or an assignment. Never, ever give up. It takes time to achieve your goals and you will most likely experience more failures than you'd like. The road will be difficult. You have to have patience and perseverance. Keep moving forward without even *thinking* about giving up. If you want something badly enough, you will go after it, regardless of how tough it is or how many setbacks you face.

Your goal in medical school is simple in this respect: Take one day at a time. Make that day as close to perfect as you can, and do not give up until you reach your goals. It's just like building a house. You do not buy all the materials and hire all the workers, then wake up the next day with a finished house. No, you wake up and use each block of time as efficiently as you can. After many months, if you don't stop building the frame, laying the bricks, putting up the drywall, and painting the walls (to name just a few steps), you will have a finished house.

Be Determined

As mentioned in the previous section, there are several types of salespeople: one who sits down passively, waiting for the opportunity to arrive, and perhaps initiating the sales pitch once, then giving up if the answer is no; the other one keeps fighting until someone actually purchases the product or service they are selling. The same principle applies to your studies and anything else you want to achieve. You can be someone who gives up after a failure or you could be so determined that you keep fighting until you've reached your goal. This example is not meant to categorize people in black and white terms. It's simply meant to demonstrate one principle of never giving up.

Consider the last type of salesperson. What was his secret? What did he do that was so special? Nothing more than being stubborn and not giving up until he made the sale. His goal was that, at the end of the day, he needed to have made X dollars, and he was not willing to take no for an answer. This is exactly how you should be. You should be determined, hard-working, and never give up until you have reached your goal. Determined people typically get what they want in the end, be it a grade, getting into medical school, getting a residency training position, or any other professional or personal success.

The Physiology of Giving Up

Every now and then, you will end up in situations where you want to give up. It can be tempting to quit when a challenge feels insurmountable. Giving up can offer you a sense of relief and control: since you will no longer be required to struggle, it can be tempting to throw in the towel[1,2]. However, the relief is very short term, and you will have to pay a higher price in the long run of giving up on your dreams and goals. There is really only one advantage of giving up: in the moment, it feels like the easiest thing to do. Otherwise, there are mostly disadvantages.

Physiologically, a critical phase in goal endeavoring occurs when multiple setbacks emerge and goal disengagement becomes a problem. This critical phase is conceptualized as an action crisis and is likely due to an internal physiological conflict in which you become torn between further goal pursuit and goal disengagement[1]. What this means in plain terms is that setbacks and challenges increase the risk that you will give up on your goals.

College and medical school are not "rocket science" designed only for geniuses. College and medical school are constructed so that the many students who get accepted can succeed if they are willing to work hard. Sure, medical school can be tough and overwhelming at times, but it is doable for most. However, finishing medical school successfully will never happen if you are passive and mentally weak. Going to school and getting good grades is hard. Very few students enjoy getting up early in the morning, coming home late in the day, and studying every day for several years. It requires ongoing effort, determination, and discipline. At the same time, there will be many distractions in your environment, some of which will be very tempting. Therefore, you need to be aware of how to minimize distractions, accept that medical school will be tough, and keep moving forward regardless of how hard it gets.

Reading hundreds of pages of a textbook, understanding the content, memorizing different terms and processes, and solving problems are demanding processes that require major effort and focus. But every year, people still manage to do it. And if they can do it, then so can you. What distinguishes those who succeed is that they are determined to reach their goals and never give up, even when it gets hard. Quite frankly, there are many things that will be hard in life, and you may have already experienced some of them, but we have to somehow manage to get through these challenges anyway.

Everyone's brain is structured in the same way. It can store memories, store new impressions, understand contexts, draw logical conclusions, and much more[3]. So, if you think about it, your brain is built in roughly the same way that Einstein's brain was. The difference lies in how you spend your time. Some understand the value of spending a lot of time on something that give them high returns later, while many others do not. Laziness is one of the biggest reasons people give up. So, set a goal that is extremely important to you and rid yourself of your inclination of ever giving up—it will never take you anywhere!

Bad Planning Increases the Risk of Giving Up

Students usually give up when their studies overwhelm them. But it's not the studies that overwhelm the students but rather bad planning. Make sure to avoid this outcome yourself by planning and prioritizing correctly. Read Chapter 6 on time management so that you can learn how to plan your studies effectively. Be sure to start studying far in advance so that your work doesn't pile up. Take control of your studies and be organized. Once you have control, you have power, and when you have power, it is your own rules that apply.

Putting Your Challenges in Perspective

You are lucky to live in a country that provides nearly everyone with the opportunity to be educated. You do not have to look far to find those who have far less "luck" than you have. Many people around the world do not have the privilege or opportunity to attend college or medical school. Instead, they must focus their efforts on daily survival. Consider how fortunate you are that you do not need to worry about meeting your basic needs, something that many of us take for granted. If you've made it to medical school, then hopefully you don't need to worry about accessing clean water or keeping a roof over your head. You also are not facing a future where your best or only option is to work 16-hour days in a dangerous factory for a few measly dollars. All you have to do is show up at school, study, and take care of yourself. Every time you feel that things are too hard or that you're ready to pack it in, put your challenges in perspective. You have it so much better than you think. And if you are struggling for any reason, there are resources available in medical school to help you.

Strategies to Never Give Up

Giving up is a biological defense mechanism that we use to lower the pressure, anxiety, and stress when we encounter a setback. As I've reminded you countless times, medical school *will* be hard. I remember many occasions when I was tired, sleep deprived, had to deal with people that were not always nice, and thought to myself, "It would be nice to just give up." And you will likely feel that way too. Many times. However, it is in these situations that you need to ask yourself, "What am I gaining if I quit now?" You have already put a lot of time and effort into this endeavor, and you know the value of your goals. So, if you give up now, you've not only wasted your time, but you will lose the benefits of all the progress you made.

Sometimes, students come up to me and say, "I have had it and I can't do this anymore—I want to cry". I always say, "Cry! It's okay to cry, but don't cry and quit! Cry and move on!" You've already come this far, so keep going and enjoy your rewards at the end!

Below I describe several strategies for you to use when you feel like giving up[4].

ADOPT AN "I WON'T QUIT" MENTALITY

This is step one. Some people won't ever give up. Read it again: They just *won't* give up. It doesn't matter how hard it gets, how many setbacks they have, how bad the worst days are. It doesn't matter. They will never, ever give up. They will never quit until they reach their goals. Continuously tell yourself the following:

- I persist when things get rough.
- I will either find a way or make one.
- There is a solution to every single problem, and I am capable of finding it.
- Every day, I gain more insight and knowledge about what works and what doesn't, which means I'm getting stronger and wiser.
- Pain is temporary.
- Setbacks are temporary.
- I will find my way through this.

WATCH OTHER PEOPLE PERSEVERE

There are many people in the world who have taken the path you are about to embark on. You can learn a lot from watching and modeling other people. There are great films, biographies, and documentaries about people who have faced incredible adversity but nonetheless refused to quit and succeeded against all odds. Learning about their stories will inspire you when you feel like giving up.

TALK TO YOUR MENTOR

In your lowest moment, it can help to talk to someone who knows you. Someone wiser and more knowledgeable than you. Someone that has walked a similar difficult path of success and knows that the feeling of wanting to quit is normal whenever you aim to achieve big things. So, call your mentor, a close friend, or someone you know who gives good advice and tell them how you're feeling.

GO BACK TO YOUR "WHY"

Whenever you feel like giving up, go back to your original reasons for starting on this path in the first place. Why did you want to reach the goal you have set for yourself? One of the most important steps in goal setting is to create a list of all the reasons why you want to achieve that goal. At the end of the day, your "why" will motivate you to continue striving, even when the road gets tough. Consequently, look at your list of reasons and if you need to, add a few more that you didn't include the first time around. The more reasons you have, and the stronger these reasons, the more likely it is that you won't quit.

RESTRATEGIZE

Another major reason why we often feel like giving up is because we repeatedly fail in our efforts. If your current approach is not working, then you need to restrategize and try a different approach. As you've probably heard before, "insanity is doing the same thing over and over again, but expecting different results." (Fun fact: Many widely believe that these words were uttered by Einstein;

in fact, these words belong to fictional character "Jane Fulton" in *Sudden Death*, a 1983 mystery novel by Rita Mae Brown.)

FAILURE IS GOOD FOR YOU

Never forget that failure has its upside. It is only when you fail that you learn new things, gain more knowledge, and become wiser. When, not if, you fail as you try to achieve your goal, then instead of using the failure as an excuse to quit, use it as a stepping stone. Tell yourself that it is *good* for you and that you can get up, restrategize if you need to, and try once again.

IT WILL BE WORTH IT IN THE END

You have goals for a reason. Becoming a physician, doing what you love, working in your chosen specialty, having financial freedom, buying the things you want, and whatever else motivates you—these are all things that will be worth the effort one day. That day, you will wake up and think back on everything you have been through. You will see how all the things that happened to you helped to make you the person you became. This is one of the fundamental truths in life: although it might be hard to appreciate and accept in the beginning, the journey matters just as much as the end result. And the harder the journey, the sweeter the victory! The challenges you endure and prevail against are what define you and help you grow. You will wake up one day and realize that you're a different type of person. Your spirit will have changed.

Pursuing a dream involves receiving a reward, perhaps long into the future. It may mean abandoning certain (bad) habits. It may mean enduring hardships. It may lead you to disappointment. But however costly it may be, going after your dream is never as high as the price paid by those who didn't live their dreams at all.

I encourage you to read this chapter from time to time or whenever you feel like giving up.

Summary

- The words "overnight success" and "medical school" do not belong in the same sentence. Success in medical school results from many good habits and working hard for many years.
- In order to succeed, you must cultivate the mentality of never giving up. The process is going to be hard, and there will be many days where you will feel exhausted, tired, and stressed out, but you just need to accept that that's the way it is and keep moving forward.
- Giving up is easy but has long-term consequences. Before you give up, you have to assess whether you are willing to accept all the consequences.
- Setbacks, challenges, and failure increase the risk that you will give up on your goals. Accept that facing obstacles and failing on occasion is a natural part of the process.
- Bad planning increases the risk of giving up, so make sure you plan well!
- Put your current circumstances and challenges in perspective; you will realize that your situation is not that bad after all.
- Strategies to not giving up include understanding the process of success (i.e., it *will* be hard work); acceptance; adopting an "I won't quit" mentality; watching others persevere; talking to mentors; reminding yourself of your "why"; restrategizing; finding the opportunity in failure; and knowing that all the effort will be worth it in the end.

References

1. Brandstätter V, Herrmann M, Schüler J. The struggle of giving up personal goals: affective, physiological, and cognitive consequences of an action crisis. *Pers Soc Psychol Bull.* 2013;39(12):1668–1682. https://doi.org/10.1177/0146167213500151.

2. Salminen ER. A guest editorial. Don't give up, don't ever give up: success is a choice. *Obstet Gynecol Surv.* 2003;58(12):791–793. https://doi.org/10.1097/01.ogx.0000097780.43905.18.

3. Maldonado KA, Alsayouri K. *Physiology, Brain.* StatPearls.com. https://www.ncbi.nlm.nih.gov/books/NBK551718/. Updated May 24, 2020.

4. Fabrega M. How to not give up—8 strategies for not quitting. Daring to Live Fully Blog. https://daringto-livefully.com/how-to-not-give-up. Accessed September 28, 2020.

CHAPTER 14

Stress Management in Medical School and How to Build a Healthy Lifestyle

Worry is like a rocking chair: it gives you something to do but never gets you anywhere.
Erma Bombeck

It is not the load that breaks you down; it's the way you carry it.
Lou Holtz

Introduction

In medical school, studying is a lifestyle. However, this lifestyle doesn't just involve reading books, attending lectures, and writing exams. You also need to ensure that all the other aspects of your life work for you, too. It's important to maintain your physical and mental health, because a strong body and mind are crucial to achieving your goals.

What we refer to as "life" is complex. Every day, your body does things involuntarily, without your conscious awareness: your lungs expand and contract, your heart circulates blood, your brain filters thousands of pieces of information. These activities occur without any effort on our part, and we often think that everything is working fine as long as we do not feel sick. But the truth is that your body has many compensatory mechanisms, meaning that it takes a long time for damage to accumulate that is either "visible" or "felt." That is why people are more prone to getting cancer or cardiovascular disease as they age: the "compensatory" defense mechanisms eventually fail. Your body can no longer fight against whichever disease process has taken hold and you start to experience symptoms.

If you are already taking care of yourself through stress management, regular exercise, a healthy diet, and adequate sleep, then you're on the right track. If you are not, then this chapter will give you guidance on how to live a healthier life. You will also want to pay attention to scientific and medical research that advises us on how we can take better care of ourselves. For example, if you are tired in the morning, then there are tips on how to be more alert. If you have trouble concentrating at times, you can significantly improve your concentration with a healthier lifestyle. All you have to do is take care of your mind and body a little better.

What is Stress?

Most students know what stress is. Most of us have felt stressed at different points in our lives, especially when we were in school. Stress is a highly subjective experience, but it is widely understood to be a "state of mental or emotional strain or tension resulting from adverse or very demanding circumstances[1]." The source of these demands can be relationships, work, finances, or school.

From a physiological perspective, the stress response is the body's natural way to defend itself against danger. Many different hormones, particularly cortisol, adrenaline, and noradrenaline, get released in the body when you feel threatened. These hormones prepare your body to confront the danger ahead facing you[1-3]. In other words, stress sends us into fight-or-flight mode. Your heart rate goes up, as does your blood pressure. You become more alert, start sweating, and get tense muscles. These physiological responses improve your ability to fight (or escape) a real danger or a challenging situation[1-3].

Over a few million years, the stress response system evolved as a way to protect us from predators. In the case of real danger to those early hunter–gatherers, such as a predator, the stress response allowed us to either fight or run away. However, nowadays we are rarely hunted by predators. Instead, the stress you or I experience is brought on by both external and internal stressors in our environment[1-3].

Different Types of Stress

Stress can be categorized in many different ways, and below are the most important types of stress for you to know about[4,5]:

- **Acute stress.** The most common form of stress, acute stress occurs on when you think about past, current, or future events. Future demands that might cause you acute stress in medical school include exams, new rotations, applications, and so on. The symptoms of acute stress are most often tension, anxiety, headache, and upset stomach. This type of stress is short term.
- **Episodic stress.** This type of stress occurs when you experience acute stress frequently. Those who are juggling many obligations and worry too much on an ongoing basis can experience episodic stress. In fact, this type of stress is common in medical school, as you will face multiple competing deadlines, exams, and other school-related obligations on a continuous basis. Episodic stress can become chronic, leading to high blood pressure and other serious consequences, such as heart disease.
- **Chronic stress.** This is the most dangerous form of stress and something I hope you never experience. If it goes on long enough, episodic stress can turn into chronic stress. Traumatic experiences such as an unhealthy or abusive relationship, a dysfunctional family, or the death of a loved one can also lead to chronic stress. Chronic stress can be subtle and often goes unnoticed because a person's coping mechanisms become a part of their personality. Studies

also show that chronic stress makes a person more prone to chronic disease. The purpose of this chapter is to give you the tools and resources to manage stress and prevent it from taking over your life.

Symptoms of Stress

Stress manifests itself in many different ways. Some stress symptoms occur in the acute phase, while others are seen in the chronic phase. Box 14.1 contains a comprehensive list of stress symptoms; however, there are a few things to keep in mind. One, you can experience any of these symptoms without experiencing stress, and two, you do not need to experience all of these symptoms in order to be considered stressed[3-5]. One or more of these symptoms can be stress related. They can lead to burnout, drug and alcohol abuse, bad eating habits, angry outburst, social withdrawal, chronic anxiety, crying, and issues with work, school, or relationships[4,5].

As you read about these symptoms, understand that experiencing them is not easy on the body and they do affect your daily living and encounters with people. If you have any of these symptoms *and* you know that a certain situation in your life is the cause of your stress, then the best strategy is to lessen or eliminate the stressor. The next-best approach is to learn about the different strategies for managing stress. That way, if you do experience acute or episodic stress, you can quickly resolve the situation.

The Importance of Recovery

Athletes know all about the need for a recovery period to rest, grow, and improve. They cannot just practice day in and day out because their bodies cannot handle it. During the recovery period is when the body adapts to the stress of exercise, replenishes its energy stores, and repairs damaged tissues[6]. It is also when muscles grow, rebuild, and strengthen. An athlete who works out too soon after intense physical exertion risks serious injury[6].

The same goes for your brain. Even though studying does not require much physical labor, all that reading, thinking, and memorization in medical school is cognitively demanding. If you do not follow proper recovery strategies, you could burn out very easily. We need to make time for

---

BOX 14.1 ■ Common Symptoms of Stress

- Headache
- Stomachache
- Cramps
- Anxiety
- Sweating
- Dizziness
- Difficulty sleeping
- Twitching
- Muscle aches
- Anger
- Difficulty focusing
- Fatigue
- Forgetfulness
- Sadness
- Restlessness
- Irritability
- Increased susceptibility to infections

both rest and recovery. That is simply how our bodies work. Even though you could potentially spend an entire month studying every day until 2 am and waking up at 6 am to go to school, your body would experience enormous strain and you would eventually burn out. Pushing yourself too hard leads to reduced productivity, poor focus, reduced capacity to memorize, difficulty sleeping, anxiety, and many other symptoms.

The fact is, you cannot ignore your fundamental biology: you need to sleep, you need to eat a healthy diet, and you need to be physically active. And the more you prioritize basic self-care, the better you will perform at school and the more you will accomplish. Most students cut back on sleep, eat poorly, and skip out on physical activity in the name of getting more studying done, not realizing that if they were to just add these things to their schedules, their results would be so much better. With that said, here are several strategies to manage stress and avoid burnout. Put these strategies into practice today and plan to implement throughout your school life.

Strategies for Stress Management

You likely already understand that being a student means experiencing stress more often than not. As I explained earlier, you needn't worry, because humans have evolved systems that help us respond to stress. It isn't realistic to expect stress to completely disappear from your life. Stress is not something you should run away from, but instead something you should be continuously mindful of, regardless of whether you feel stressed at this very moment.

Here is where self-awareness comes into play. Begin to pay more attention to what situations or factors make you feel more stressed as well as what symptoms you tend to experience under stress. Next, get ready to learn a variety of relaxation techniques and healthy lifestyle practices that will help you feel your best.

RELAXATION TECHNIQUES

Relaxation techniques are one of the most effective tools for stress management. However, most students do not prioritize relaxation because of their workloads. The truth is that everyone needs to relax and recharge so that the body can repair itself. Relaxation techniques not only help you to reduce stress, but they also increase your productivity, improve your focus and attention, and enhance your overall health and well-being[7].

MEDITATION

I'm sure you've heard it before, but I'll say it again: meditation is an extremely powerful habit to cultivate. Done the right way and done consistently, it can benefit you significantly. Many studies have shown that meditation changes the structure of and increases blood flow to the brain; reduces cortisol, blood pressure, and heart rate; increases neuroplasticity; releases serotonin and dopamine (two neurotransmitters that make you feel happier); boosts your immune system; promotes muscle relaxation[8-13]. Meditation can also reduce feelings of anxiety and depression. Regular meditation also makes you more resistant to stress, increases your positive emotions and emotional stability; improves your focus and moment-to-moment awareness; increases your emotional stability; and even increases your capacity to learn[8-13]. Doesn't this all sound great? Then why doesn't everyone do it? Good question.

One of the reasons that meditation is a difficult practice to turn into a regular habit is that these effects do not come right away. In fact, the positive benefits of meditation accrue over time. Sometimes a really long time. You have to consistently meditate for weeks and months if not years! Since it takes such a long time to derive these benefits, and since there appear to be no immediate, noticeable, and positive effects, many try it a few times and then quit.

My recommendation is that you find a good meditation program with a teacher whose voice you like, stick to the program, and consistently do your meditation. Try to wake up 10 to 15 minutes before your regular wake-up time and do it first thing the morning. Even 10 minutes a day will make a big difference in the long run. I promise that you will feel a change if you do it regularly and give it time. Make meditation one of your daily habits, just like your brushing your teeth.

YOGA

With so many different types of yoga classes to choose from, it's likely that you've tried yoga at least once in your life. If not, it's worth giving it a try: yoga is a great form of stress relief. You can try different types of yoga until you find the one that's right for you and your personality. Postural yoga, the main type of yoga practiced in the United States, strengthens and stretches the body and focuses on using the breath to relax the mind and body. Yoga classes also frequently include a period of meditation. At home, you can do a yoga practice in as little as 10 to 20 minutes a day.

Yoga continues to be the subject of much scientific research. A systematic review of 14 studies that examined the effects of yoga on the body concluded that it has the following significant positive benefits[14]:

- Reduces stress
- Increases energy
- Lowers blood pressure and heart rate
- Improves respiration
- Reduces anxiety and depression, and
- Reduces physiological arousal.

CUTTING BACK ON STIMULANTS

When a person is stressed, it is easy to reach for stimulants such as alcohol, drugs, and nicotine[15]. Unfortunately, these substances do not help to prevent or reduce stress; in fact, they can actually make you feel worse. While they might calm you down temporarily, your stress symptoms will return a short time later, after the stimulant leaves your body[15]. Therefore, do your best to cut back on or eliminate their use.

TALKING

When you are worried, stressed, and not feeling well in general, it helps to talk it out with someone. And not just talk it out one time but several times and perhaps with different people who have different perspectives[16]. You should never go it alone with your problems. Talk to family, friends, and mentors and vent about what's troubling you. I promise you that it will not only help you feel better, but you may also get a lot of tips from others who have been in your shoes[16]. You will also see that you are not the only one who feels the way you feel. If you are feeling incredibly agitated and have one or more prolonged symptoms of stress, then please be sure to see a doctor.

POSITIVE THINKING

Positive thinking helps[17,18]! Your thoughts and beliefs about yourself and your life circumstances can shape the outcome of events. Go back and look at your goals, dreams, and plans. Think about your future and look at your resources. There is always a way to solve a problem. It's important to take control and feel that you have agency. One way to do this is to think positive, remember who you are and what you're capable of, and keep your goals and dreams foremost in your mind. Moreover, think about past obstacles you have encountered and successfully overcome. When you reframe your situation and remind yourself that you are capable of finding a solution, your thoughts will change and you'll get back on track.

PHYSICAL ACTIVITY

The importance of engaging in physical activity is a message that is hammered into us on a daily basis. Physical activity makes for better physical *and* mental health[19-23]. Whatever you have tended do in your spare time until today, things are about to change: from now on, make sure that you make time for *at least* two workouts per week. If you can do four or five workouts per week, even better.

There has been extensive research on the benefits of physical activity. So the sooner you get moving, the better. People who exercise regularly are healthier and are able to use their physical and mental capacity more effectively than others[19-23]. Box 14.2 details just some of the many positive effects that you can experience when you exercise regularly[19-23]. These positive effects relate directly to your life as a student and will undoubtedly help you with your studies.

I understand that you have a crazy schedule (I've been there), but that is no excuse for not exercising just a couple of times a week. Working out should be as natural as, you guessed it, brushing your teeth. You brush your teeth because you want healthy teeth and good oral health; you wash your body to keep it clean and healthy; and you eat nutritious food to feel energized. As obvious as all those things are, many people still forget to include weekly or daily exercise. Remember that exercising just a few times a week will only improve your sleep quality, energy, stress level, and ultimately school performance[19-23].

When you exercise, you reduce the stress hormones in your body and increase the level of endorphins. This in turn gives you that natural boost of happy hormones and energy that you need in between hard study sessions[19-23]. Physical activity also distracts your mind from negative thoughts, which tend to be more common when you are feeling stressed out by your studies. Many of us also enjoy listening to music while we exercise. Music is something that makes us feel good and has its own benefits[19-23].

After a long study session, you will probably feel tense and tired. The perfect cure for the lethargy and tension you feel is to head to the gym or go for a run. It doesn't really matter what you do as long as it's something that elevates your heart rate for 30 minutes. You can cycle, play football, run, do aerobics, or dance. The important thing is to do *something* that gives your brain a break from studying. Then you can return to your studies with renewed energy and increased focus. I have friends that say that if they do NOT work out, they feel lousy and cannot focus at all. So keep

---

BOX 14.2 ■ Benefits of Regular Physical Activity

- Improved performance
- Improved learning ability and memory
- More energy
- Better sleep
- Reduced stress, anxiety, and depression
- Stronger immune system (less chance of getting sick)
- Better posture
- Increased fitness and endurance
- Improved oxygen uptake
- Reduced risk for cardiovascular disease
- Reduced risk for certain cancers
- Reduced risk of dying prematurely

that in mind when you consider skipping a trip to the gym to study for an extra hour. You'll get a lot more out of moving your body and working up a sweat. Physical activity—not watching TV or scrolling through social media—is the perfect study break.

Finally, remember that you need just 30 to 60 minutes of physical activity at least twice a week. There is simply no excuse for not exercising. If you schedule and prioritize physical activity, then you *will* make it happen. Just like you make studying happen.

HEALTHY DIET

The road to success in medical school takes many years, and that means you have to think of the many factors that will affect your performance other than study techniques. One of those things is diet. What you eat has a major influence on your health and is therefore another important factor in your success.

Take a moment to think about how you're currently fueling your body—would you say that your diet is a healthy one? A healthy diet is one that is rich in vitamins, minerals, and fiber and that provides you with plenty of energy without making you gain weight. Most of us have some basic knowledge of what food is classified as healthy (nutritious) versus unhealthy (lacking in nutrients). But it's more complicated than that. Because nutrition affects so many aspects of your health, now is the time to assess the quality of your diet and learn more about how what you eat affects your mental and physical performance. You will notice how much better you feel both physically and mentally once you switch to healthier eating habits. The healthier the food, the better your health and ability to perform well in school.

What to Eat

First, let's discuss "fast" and "slow" carbohydrates, which refers to how quickly your blood sugar increases when you eat different foods. If you eat a chocolate bar, for instance, you will notice that you become energized almost immediately, which is the result of a spike in your blood sugar. However, soon after you will feel hungry and irritable and have difficulty concentrating, a sign that your blood sugar has gone back down. The problem with fast carbohydrates such as sweets, chocolates, and white bread is that both the spike and the crash in your blood sugar happen very quickly, which in turn negatively affects your focus and makes you tired. Fast carbohydrates are not a stable source of energy.

By comparison, slow carbohydrates such as beans, whole grains, and nuts cause your blood sugar to rise and fall more slowly. Your blood sugar is kept steady for a longer period of time, which in turn gives you more sustained energy. Therefore, when putting together your meals for the day, your aim should be to keep your blood sugar as even as possible by eating more slow carbohydrates. Not only are slow carbohydrates much better for you, they also increase your focus and performance.

To get an idea of which carbohydrates are fast and slow, it helps to know about the glycemic index of different foods. A food with a glycemic index over 70 or 80, such as white bread and various sweets, is considered a fast carbohydrate; it does not provide you with a consistent blood sugar level. Foods with a glycemic index of 60 or below are slow carbohydrates; these are the foods you should be eating more of to ensure a steady energy level throughout the day. You can search for glycemic index tables online to learn more about the foods you eat.

With regard to what to eat specifically, that is more complex and a whole book in itself, if not 10 books. There are a lot of books and scientific papers on different diets for specific needs, but we will not go into that. However, there are two diets that in multiple trials have been shown to have the greatest health benefits for the average person, at least with respect to preventing chronic diseases: the Mediterranean diet and the Dietary Approaches to Stop Hypertension (DASH) diet. Many diets promise weight loss, so if that is your primary aim, then you should look up an eating plan that will help you lose weight. Nonetheless, my primary aim here is that you eat a healthy diet that prevents major chronic illnesses. Therefore, we will focus on the Mediterranean diet, as the DASH diet focuses on lowering high blood pressure.

The Mediterranean diet emphasizes eating plant foods and healthy fats to reduce the risk of heart disease. More evidence is emerging that this diet also provides other benefits like preserving your memory. The Mediterranean diet first received close attention when researchers learned that people living in the Mediterranean region had a lower incidence and prevalence of cardiovascular disease; researchers concluded that their diet must have something to do with that, both what they ate and did not eat.

The Mediterranean diet consists mainly of the following foods:

- Plants, including vegetables, fruits, nuts, legumes, and whole grains
- Olive oil as the main source of fat
- Moderate amount of fish and poultry
- No or very small amounts of red meat
- No or very small amounts of sweets, and
- Small to moderate amounts of wine.

The PREDIMED study, to date the largest dietary intervention trial to assess the effects of the Mediterranean diet, involved nearly 7,500 people in Spain aged 55 to 80 years. Researchers found that the group eating the Mediterranean diet had 30% less chance of heart attack, stroke, or other heart disease–related etiologies[24,25]. Other trials have also shown the benefits of the Mediterranean diet[26,27]. The main gist is that you eat should a lot of salad, fish, and olive oil, preferably extra-virgin olive oil, as your main source of fat. Add some fruit and eat only a little red meat. For lunch, have a salad. As your snack between lunch and dinner, have two fruits, and for dinner try different types of fish.

The Mediterranean diet has been my diet of choice for many years. I feel energized, alert, and focused. In short, it makes me feel healthy. Sometimes, I will throw in a protein bar, which you can do as well. After a workout, I will make a healthy smoothie with almond milk, a scoop of protein powder, kale, strawberries, blueberries, blackberries, raspberries, turmeric, ginger, orange, and an apple. You can mix a smoothie however you want as long as you add antioxidants, fruit, and vegetables.

I am also not saying that you can never enjoy a burger or pizza. I enjoy those too, and I think eating junk food once in a while is part of quality of life. But as long as you're not making it a daily habit to eat junk food, you need not worry.

Breakfast remains controversial. People used to say that breakfast was the most important meal of the day; however, many do not believe that this is the case anymore. In fact, new studies show that fasting for several hours is very good for the body and can reduce inflammation; improve blood sugar control by reducing insulin resistance; boost brain function such as focus and performance; reduce weight; and extend longevity, among other benefits[28-31].

There are different types of fasting, but the one I do is intermittent fasting for 12 to 16 hours. I typically have my last meal around 8 or 9 pm and then will not eat anything else until lunch the next day. I drink plenty of water and black coffee in the morning and that's it. This works for me and may not work for you, but studies show that intermittent fasting can be beneficial. Furthermore, if you're usually in a rush in the mornings and want to sleep in a bit more, intermittent fasting could be a great approach for you.

SLEEP

Both quality and length of sleep are important. Many students do not prioritize sleep as they should because they underestimate its importance. I have known plenty of students who would rather study an extra 2 or 3 hours a night and get only 2 or 3 hours of sleep. A couple of times per month can be okay, but long-term sleep deprivation will negatively affect you. New guidelines show that an adult needs 7 to 9 hours of sleep per night[32,33]. Before these new guidelines were announced, adults were recommended to sleep a minimum of 6 hours per night, but research found that those who sleep an average of 6 hours are at increased risk of chronic health issues[32,33].

Here are a few of the many important reasons why you should get enough sleep[34]:

- **Memory and learning.** People who get more sleep learn and remember tasks better. Sleep helps the brain store memories more effectively.
- **General health.** Sleep deprivation has been linked to many chronic health conditions such as high blood pressure, heart arrhythmias, and increased stress hormone levels.
- **Mood.** Sleep deprivation can lead to impatience, poor focus, irritability, and moodiness.
- **Immune system.** A lack of sleep affects your immune system and can make you more susceptible to colds and infections.
- **Metabolism.** Sleep helps to control your metabolism; those who do not sleep enough are at greater risk of gaining weight.

With this basic knowledge, you should now understand that, if you haven't already, you need to implement a healthy sleep regimen. Studies show that you cannot go without sleep for days on end and then just "make up for it" in one night or weekend[34]. The best sleeping habit is the one that is consistent.

Here are some sleep tips for you to follow to get a good night's sleep[35,36]:

- Get at least 7 hours of sleep and not more than 9 hours.
- Keep a consistent sleep schedule wherever you go. Go to bed and wake up at around the same time every day as much as possible.
- If you cannot fall asleep after 20 minutes, get out of bed and do something else for 5 to 10 minutes such as reading a book or making a cup of herbal tea, then try to go to sleep again. Do not use your phone or log into your computer.
- Create a relaxing environment that is conducive to sleep. Your bedroom should be quiet and cool at night with limited light exposure. Get a good mattress and pillow, and don't keep electronics by the bedside.
- Avoid eating a large meal right before bed.
- Avoid caffeine or alcohol consumption a few hours before bed.
- Use your bedroom mostly for sleep.

If you aren't already sleeping well, then following these healthy sleep habits consistently will help you get your sleep hygiene and consequently health back on the right track.

HOBBIES AND ENTERTAINMENT

Remember to have something of a life outside school and studying. You cannot just study day in and out without taking breaks and doing something fun or enjoyable. While I have emphasized the importance of studying and working hard, you do still need to have hobbies and enjoy life. A life without fun in between all the hard work will soon become very frustrating and perhaps even disabling for you. Hobbies are an important part of mental health and wellness, as they will support you by offering you a rewarding social outlet and stimulate your brain in a way that studying cannot[37-40]. Hobbies bring a sense of fun and can make you look forward to things when your life seem tedious and difficult. Hobbies help to reduce stress and boost your brain function. It makes *you* more interesting too, as you will have stories and experiences to share with others; they also make you more patient with learning new things[37-40]. Hobbies also improve your confidence and boost your self-esteem. They eradicate boredom, increase your knowledge, challenge you, and help you develop new skills[37-40]. Most importantly, hobbies offer you a temporary and healthy "escape" from a potentially stressful environment from time to time.

It doesn't really matter what your hobby is. The important thing is that you find one or several that you can do consistently. If you do not have any hobbies, get out there and explore: try painting, dancing, rock climbing, cooking, singing, or gardening. You might think that having a hobby is a waste of time, but I am telling you that you must have other things to do in life besides studying.

The same goes with entertainment. When you're in medical school, it's not reasonable to watch TV and play on your computer day and night. But if you really do enjoy a certain show or video game, then doing that for 30 to 60 minutes a few times per week when you have some time is okay. You may want to spend time with your friends and go out one night. Again, this is totally fine and something you can do as long you are not falling behind on assignments and exams.

I used to treat myself to watching an inspiring documentary for half an hour every night. But I would only let myself do that if I had completed my to-do list and was on top of my studies. If you have a good plan, a solid study schedule, and work hard as this book will teach you, you will most likely be able to have some time for entertainment. Hobbies and entertainment are an important part of your recovery and stress management. Make a bit of time in your schedule to step away from your books each day. Treat yourself from time to time. Don't forget to live.

Summary

- In medical school, studying is a lifestyle. To make that lifestyle work for you, you will need to take care of all aspects of your health. That means ensuring you eat a healthy diet, get regular physical activity, sleep at least 6 to 7 hours every night, and have hobbies you enjoy. You should practice these healthy habits from day one of medical school.
- The stress response is the body's natural defense against a threat in its environment. Several different hormones, particularly cortisol, adrenaline, and noradrenaline, are released in the body when you feel threatened. These hormones prepare your body to confront the danger facing you.
- Three are three main types of stress: acute, episodic, and chronic. Chronic stress poses the most danger to your long-term health.
- Symptoms of stress include headache, cramps, stomachache, anxiety, sweating, dizziness, sleep issues, anger, fatigue, forgetfulness, sadness, and irritability.
- Recovery from hard work and stress is important.
- Use the stress management techniques and advice contained in this chapter to learn how to better manage your stress and avoid the lasting harm of chronic stress.

References

1. McEwen BS. Physiology and neurobiology of stress and adaptation: central role of the brain. *Physiol Rev.* 2007;87(3):873–904. https://doi.org/10.1152/physrev.00041.2006.
2. Yaribeygi H, Panahi Y, Sahraei H, Johnston TP, Sahebkar A. The impact of stress on body function: a review. *EXCLI J.* 2017;16:1057–1072. https://doi.org/10.17179/excli2017-480.
3. Mariotti A. The effects of chronic stress on health: new insights into the molecular mechanisms of brain-body communication. *Future Sci OA.* 2015;1(3):FSO23. https://doi.org/10.4155/fso.15.21.
4. Everything You Need to Know About Stress. https://www.healthline.com/health/stress#hormones.
5. Ehrenfeld T. Three Types of Stress. Psychology Today. https://www.psychologytoday.com/us/blog/opengently/201812/the-three-types-stress. Published December 7, 2018.
6. Crespo-Ruiz B, Rivas-Galan S, Fernandez-Vega C, Crespo-Ruiz C, Maicas-Perez L. Executive stress management: physiological load of stress and recovery in executives on workdays. *Int J Environ Res Public Health.* 2018;15(12):2847. https://doi.org/10.3390/ijerph15122847.
7. Mayo Clinic. *Stress Management—Relaxation Techniques.* https://www.mayoclinic.org/healthy-lifestyle/stress-management/basics/relaxation-techniques/hlv-20049495. Published March 21, 2020.

8. Chen KW, Berger CC, Manheimer E, et al. Meditative therapies for reducing anxiety: a systematic review and meta-analysis of randomized controlled trials. *Depression Anxiety.* 2012;29(7):545–562. https://doi.org/10.1002/da.21964.

9. Clarke TC, Barnes PM, Black LI, Stussman BJ, Nahin RL. *Use of yoga, meditation, and chiropractors among U.S. adults aged 18 and over.* NCHS Data Brief No. 325. Hyattsville, MD: National Center for Health Statistics; 2018.

10. Dakwar E, Levin FR. The emerging role of meditation in addressing psychiatric illness, with a focus on substance use disorders. *Harv Rev Psychiatry.* 2009;17(4):254–267. https://doi.org/10.1080/10673220903149135.

11. Desbordes G, Negi LT, Pace TW, et al. Effects of mindful-attention and compassion meditation training on amygdala response to emotional stimuli in an ordinary, non-meditative state. *Front Hum Neurosci.* 2012;6:1–15. https://doi.org/10.3389/fnhum.2012.00292.

12. Fang CY, Reibel DK, Longacre ML, et al. Enhanced psychosocial well-being following participation in a mindfulness-based stress reduction program is associated with increased natural killer cell activity. *J Altern Complement Med.* 2010;16(5):531–538. https://doi.org/10.1089/acm.2009.0018.

13. Goyal M, Singh S, Sibinga EM, et al. Meditation programs for psychological stress and well-being: a systematic review and meta-analysis. *JAMA Inter Med.* 2014;174(3):357–368. https://doi.org/10.1001/jamainternmed.2013.13018.

14. Domingues RB. Modern postural yoga as a mental health promoting tool: a systematic review. *Complement Ther Clin Pract.* 2018 May;31:248–255. https://doi.org/10.1016/j.ctcp.2018.03.002.

15. Sinha R. Chronic stress, drug use, and vulnerability to addiction. *Ann N Y Acad Sci.* 2008;1141:105–130. https://doi.org/10.1196/annals.1441.030.

16. Keegan L. Therapies to reduce stress and anxiety. *Crit Care Nurs Clin North Am.* 2003;15(3):321–327. https://doi.org/10.1016/s0899-5885(02)00103-x.

17. Eagleson C, Hayes S, Mathews A, Perman G, Hirsch CR. The power of positive thinking: pathological worry is reduced by thought replacement in generalized anxiety disorder. *Behav Res Ther.* 2016;78:13–18. https://doi.org/10.1016/j.brat.2015.12.017.

18. Motamed-Jahromi M, Fereidouni Z, Dehghan A. Effectiveness of positive thinking training program on nurses' quality of work life through smartphone applications. *Int Sch Res Notices.* 2017;2017. https://doi.org/10.1155/2017/4965816.

19. Warburton DE, Nicol CW, Bredin SS. Health benefits of physical activity: the evidence. *CMAJ.* 2006;174(6):801–809. https://doi.org/10.1503/cmaj.051351.

20. Bauman AE. Updating the evidence that physical activity is good for health: an epidemiological review 2000–2003. *J Sci Med Sport.* 2004;7(1 Suppl):6–19. https://doi.org/10.1016/s1440-2440(04)80273-1.

21. Tseng CN, Gau BS, Lou MF. The effectiveness of exercise on improving cognitive function in older people: a systematic review. *J Nurs Res.* 2011;19(2):119–131. https://doi.org/10.1097/JNR.0b013e3182198837.

22. Bize R, Johnson JA, Plotnikoff RC. Physical activity level and health-related quality of life in the general adult population: a systematic review. *Prev Med.* 2007;45(6):401–415. https://doi.org/10.1016/j.ypmed.2007.07.017.

23. Gerber M, Puhse U. Review article: do exercise and fitness protect against stress-induced health complaints? A review of the literature. *Scand J Public Health.* 2009;37(8):801–819. https://doi.org/10.1177/1403494809350522.

24. Estruch R, Ros E, Salas-Salvadó J, et al. Primary prevention of cardiovascular disease with a Mediterranean diet. *N Engl J Med.* 2013;368(14):1279–1290. https://doi.org/10.1056/NEJMoa1200303.

25. Estruch R, Ros E, Salas-Salvadó J, et al. Primary prevention of cardiovascular disease with a Mediterranean diet supplemented with extra-virgin olive oil or nuts. *N Engl J Med.* 2018;378(25):e34. https://doi.org/10.1056/NEJMoa1800389.

26. Tosti V, Bertozzi B, Fontana L. Health benefits of the Mediterranean diet: metabolic and molecular mechanisms. *J Gerontol A Biol Sci Med Sci.* 2018;73(3):318–326. https://doi.org/10.1093/gerona/glx227.

27. Martínez-González MA. Benefits of the Mediterranean diet beyond the Mediterranean Sea and beyond food patterns. *BMC Med.* 2016;14(1):157. https://doi.org/10.1186/s12916-016-0714-3.

28. Trepanowski JF, Kroeger CM, Barnosky A, et al. Effect of alternate-day fasting on weight loss, weight maintenance, and cardioprotection among metabolically healthy obese adults: a randomized clinical trial. *JAMA Intern Med.* 2017;177(7):930–938. https://doi.org/10.1001/jamainternmed.2017.0936.

29. Heilbronn LK, Smith SR, Martin CK, Anton SD, Ravussin E. Alternate-day fasting in nonobese subjects: effects on body weight, body composition, and energy metabolism. *Am J Clin Nutr.* 2005;81(1):69–73. https://doi.org/10.1093/ajcn/81.1.69.

30. Harris L, Hamilton S, Azevedo LB, et al. Intermittent fasting interventions for treatment of overweight and obesity in adults: a systematic review and meta-analysis. *JBI Database Syst Rev Implement Rep.* 2018;16(2):507–547. https://doi.org/10.11124/JBISRIR-2016-003248.

31. Sutton EF, Beyl R, Early KS, Cefalu WT, Ravussin E, Peterson CM. Early time-restricted feeding improves insulin sensitivity, blood pressure, and oxidative stress even without weight loss in men with prediabetes. *Cell Metab.* 2018;27(6). https://doi.org/10.1016/j.cmet.2018.04.010. 1212–1221.e3.

32. Watson NF, Badr MS, Belenky G, et al. Recommended amount of sleep for a healthy adult: a joint consensus statement of the American Academy of Sleep Medicine and Sleep Research Society. *Sleep.* 2015;38(6):843–844. https://doi.org/10.5665/sleep.4716.

33. Chaput JP, Dutil C, Sampasa-Kanyinga H. Sleeping hours: what is the ideal number and how does age impact this? *Nat Sci Sleep.* 2018;10:421–430. https://doi.org/10.2147/NSS.S163071.

34. Importance of sleep: six reasons not to scrimp on sleep. Harvard Health Publishing. https://www.health.harvard.edu/press_releases/importance_of_sleep_and_health. Published January 2006.

35. Institute for Quality and Efficiency in Health Care. Insomnia: relaxation techniques and sleeping habits. https://www.ncbi.nlm.nih.gov/books/NBK279320/. Published August 18, 2008. Updated March 9, 2017.

36. Yazdi Z, Loukzadeh Z, Moghaddam P, Jalilolghadr S. Sleep hygiene practices and their relation to sleep quality in medical students of Qazvin University of Medical Sciences. *J Caring Sci.* 2016;5(2):153–160. https://doi.org/10.15171/jcs.2016.016.

37. Pressman SD, Matthews KA, Cohen S, et al. Association of enjoyable leisure activities with psychological and physical well-being. *Psychosom Med.* 2009;71(7):725–732. https://doi.org/10.1097/PSY.0b013e3181ad7978.

38. Takeda F, Noguchi H, Monma T, Tamiya N. How possibly do leisure and social activities impact mental health of middle-aged adults in Japan? An evidence from a national longitudinal survey. *PLoS One.* 2015;10(10). https://doi.org/10.1371/journal.pone.0139777.

39. Willius FA. The necessity and importance of adoption of sedentary hobbies. *Proc Staff Meet Mayo Clin.* 1948;23(18):412.

40. McQuoid J. Finding joy in poor health: the leisure-scapes of chronic illness. *Soc Sci Med.* 2017;183:88–96. https://doi.org/10.1016/j.socscimed.2017.04.044.

Study Techniques

CHAPTER 15

Anatomy, Histology, and Pharmacology Courses

Introduction

Anatomy, histology, and pharmacology courses mainly require that you memorize massive amounts of information. In anatomy, for instance, you have to know the names of different structures of the human body. In histology, you have to know the name of each histological structure as well as how they look at the microscopic level. In pharmacology, you have to learn the names and functions of different drugs, how they affect the body, their side effects and interactions, and so forth.

Although there is some degree of understanding required, most of the work is pure memorization, and the learning process is virtually the same for each of the courses. Consequently, the study technique for these courses involves using different memorization methods in a structured, organized, and systematic way. For simplicity, I will illustrate how to use this study method using the anatomy course as an example. In histology, there are additional steps to do, which are noted at the end of this section.

Step by Step

1. Determine exactly what you need to learn before the exam. Find out what is expected from you in terms of the exact page numbers, tasks, and problems you need to solve. This is crucial to know, because you want to make sure you do not miss any areas for the exam.
2. Make an organized plan. Go back to Chapter 6 on time management and create a structured plan for your exam(s).
3. Start by organizing the content on each organ or body part in its own section. For instance, start with the face, then the chest, the abdomen, the liver, the heart, and so on. Let's say you are starting with the face. The important anatomical structures to learn in the face are the nerves, the muscles, the arteries, and the veins, to name a few. Organize each anatomical area on its own. For instance, start with the nerves, then the arteries, then the muscles, and so on.
4. Now that you have organized all the parts within an area of the body, it's time to start studying. Note that there are three other steps to perform before you start to study! The planning and organizing you do before your study session is critical. There will likely be multiple books, online materials, and other reading material that will be available for you to

consult. It will be impossible to read everything that you can find on each topic. Therefore, choose one or a few key resources and stick with them. Which book is best for each category or course is debatable, but I advise you to go with the book that your school has recommended for that particular area. If you have lecture notes and articles that you think are high-yield, you should certainly stick with those as well. However, do not hop from book to book and start reading 10 different resources because you won't have a good structure to your reading, and you may even get confused about the information, since different authors write in different ways. Thus, pick one or a couple of resources and stick with them. You can also ask around a few of your seniors; ask them which books they used and what feedback they can offer you.

5. Now, use the memorization and learning techniques described in Chapter 11 to read the course book(s) you have chosen, studying the content in the order you decided on in step 3. Make sure you use association, visualization, chunking, spaced repetition, and acronyms or mnemonics to learn and memorize the material.

6. As you read through each of the different areas, write down certain parts in your own words using your memorization techniques. For instance, if you are using a mnemonic to memorize the cranial nerves, write it down in an organized way. If you are making associations with different muscles, then write those down. Remember that you do not have to write down every single thing you read because that is a waste of time, especially in the beginning when everything feels new and difficult. But do write down the information that is harder for you to comprehend or remember or that requires specific memorization techniques.

7. Repetition, repetition, repetition. Remember that repetition is the key to learn anything new. Even though it won't seem to you as though you're learning much in the beginning, have patience, because it will in the end if you are stubborn enough to keep on reading the material over and over again. Thus, focus on repetition. There will be a lot of times where you feel that this will not work or that you will never learn certain things. Trust me when I say that most students go through these phases. Repeat the information over and over again. Be diligent and consistent.

8. Here is where you practice spaced repetition. Once you have read one section, go to the next section; when you have read the section on cranial nerves, go to the section on the arteries of the face. But before you go to the third section, skim through the first section again very rapidly (e.g., the section on cranial nerves), and then move on to the third section (Box 15.1).

9. Now, we have arrived at retrieval practice. This method involves describing something you have learned, to yourself, in your own words. For this step, start by recalling the different areas and connect them together.

10. Quizzes and flashcards. Once you have repeated the above steps a number of times, you should start doing quizzes, old exam, and flashcards. Put simply, you should start testing yourself with questions. This step should be done fairly early on in your study plan. Answering questions and solving problems improves not only your memory but also your understanding. Your brain starts to process the information needed to solve a problem or answer a question. At this step, you will get the chance to recall information you've read before and reinforce your memory so that you can apply your knowledge in a clinical setting. Quizzes are also good to do because the questions that are typically asked are centered around the most important aspects of the topic. Answering questions allows you to identify your weak areas early so that you can go back to those areas and study them more carefully. Therefore, quizzes should be a big part of your study strategy. Do them regularly and at an early stage.

11. You will now start learning about a new part of the body. Repeat steps 3–11.

> **BOX 15.1 ■ Step 8—Learning the Course Material Through Spaced Repetition**
>
> Let's say that you are starting to learn the nerves of the face. Once you have completed your first round of learning the nerves, you will want to study the arteries of the face, and then the veins of the face. After you've studied the arteries, and before you move onto studying the veins, skim through your notes on the nerves again as well as the arteries, and then start with your third section, the veins of the face. Remember that spaced repetition, the method of recalling the information you want to learn in expanding intervals, has been shown in scientific studies to work very effectively in remembering new knowledge[1,2].
>
> After the third section (on the veins of the face), review the fourth section. Now, before you start with the fifth section, go back to read the third and fourth sections again, and then start with the fifth section. Once you are done with the fifth section, go back and recall the first, second, third, fourth, and fifth sections again before you start with the sixth. Are you confused? Don't be; it is quite simple. Here is an outline of how to systematically do spaced repetition:
>
> 1. Read area 1.
> 2. Read area 2.
> 3. Repeat area 1.
> 4. Repeat area 2.
> 5. Read area 3.
> 6. Read area 4.
> 7. Repeat area 3.
> 8. Repeat area 4.
> 9. Read area 5.
> 10. Go back to area 1 and repeat area 1.
> 11. Repeat area 2.
> 12. Repeat area 3.
> 13. Repeat area 4.
> 14. Repeat area 5.
> 15. Start reading area 6.
> 16. Etc.
>
> Remember that you might not have six different areas or sections to study for a particular part of the body, or you might have 10 areas to study. It all depends on what you are studying. However, the study technique is the same. First, you organize the content on each part of the body. Then, you structure the content according to different areas of the anatomical structures you need to study. Finally, you start reading and reviewing the sections you have already read before you continue further to read a new section.

STEP 9—RETRIEVAL PRACTICE

Here is an example of how to do retrieval practice.

You state that the facial nerve is cranial nerve 7 and that it has five major branches in the face: the temporal/frontal branch, the zygomatic branch, the buccal branch, the marginal mandibular branch, and the cervical branch. You then continue by naming all the muscles that the different branches are innervating. When you cannot recall something, you simply look it up in your book and then move onto the next section. Continue doing the same thing for other anatomical regions.

While this method is rather time consuming, it is an effective way to learn and memorize new information. It also helps you to ensure that you are understanding the material you've read. Using this method together with other techniques allows for greater cognitive effort (more than simply rereading), which in turn results in higher levels of conceptual learning and application of the knowledge[3-5]. But remember that retrieval practice comes *after* doing a few rounds of repetition (steps 4–8); if you do this step too early in your studying, then you may have to look up too many things, which will take too much of your limited study time. Remember also that you may be very unsuccessful at recalling things in the beginning, and that is okay. It will take time for you to be able to recall everything well! But the more you do it, the better you will get at it.

Histology

The study method for histology involves similar a process to that described for anatomy and pharmacology. The only difference is that you also have to spend time learning the visual aspect of the body's tissues. Learning visual diagnosis is generally easier than learning fact-based knowledge. Seeing something and putting a name to it is considered an effective way to learn[6].

Therefore, you should not get stressed out about the fact that your histology course is going to be more difficult than your other courses. It is just a different way of learning. The visual information about the tissues is one additional layer and is quite fun to learn, since you will get to know what different organs and their cells are supposed to look like.

Start studying your histology course content by following the exact same steps as before, but with the addition of one step—the visual part of the course—in which you will learn how different tissues in the body look. Start with steps 1–4, organizing the content on each tissue type. As you read through the different areas, write down certain parts in your own words using your memorization techniques. Then go to step 5 and 6, where you will have to either learn the different tissue in the lab with a microscope or practice your visual memory of the different tissues by using the images in your textbook. The key here is to not just remember the names but also how the tissues look. Therefore, steps 5 and 6 require that you spend time memorizing and understanding what the tissues look like and connecting their visual description with the factual knowledge you have learned.

Once you are done with step 6, you can continue with steps 7, 8, and 9 as described before. In step 7, you will recall to yourself how different tissues look by explaining the different cells they have, their color, structures, and so forth. In step 8, you will go through all the sections on each type of tissue. Finally, you will quiz yourself. The quizzes should not only be factual but also give you images of different tissues and cells to identify and describe.

A few last items to note. Start early with your planning and reading. These courses can be very frustrating, since the volume of material is extremely high; it is not so hard to understand but rather simply a lot to memorize. That could make histology, for instance, a lot less fun than your other courses. However, stay motivated and be consistent. These courses are crucial and a big part of your knowledge foundation in medicine. Moreover, understand that it *will* take time to learn all of the information and that it is *not* easy. However, it is doable; if others have done it, then you can too.

References

1. Dobson JL. Effect of uniform versus expanding retrieval practice on the recall of physiology information. *Adv Physiol Educ.* 2012;36(1):6–12.
2. Storm BC, Bjork RA, Storm JC. Optimizing retrieval as a learning event: when and why expanding retrieval practice enhances long-term retention. *Mem Cognit.* 2010;38(2):244–253.
3. Kornell N, Hays MJ, Bjork RA. Unsuccessful retrieval attempts enhance subsequent learning. *J Exp Psychol Learn Mem Cogn.* 2009;35(4):989–998.
4. Sleister H. Evidence-based strategies to improve memory and learning. *J Microbiol Biol Educ.* 2014;15(2):336–337. https://doi.org/10.1128/jmbe.v15i2.790.
5. Augustin M. How to learn effectively in medical school: test yourself, learn actively, and repeat in intervals. *Yale J Biol Med.* 2014;87(2):207–212.
6. Bobek E, Tversky B. Creating visual explanations improves learning. *Cogn Res Princ Implic.* 2016;1(1):27. https://doi.org/10.1186/s41235-016-0031-6.

Biochemistry, Cell Biology, Genetics, and Biology Courses

Introduction

Biochemistry, cell biology, genetics, and biology courses tend to have one thing in common: they consist of content that must be read and understood, as well as problems that must be solved based on the content. More specifically, you will be tested on your ability to (1) comprehend the different chemical and biological processes in the cell and (2) apply this knowledge to solving problems. Some memorization of information is involved, but mostly you should focus your efforts on understanding the content. The ability to problem solve and apply concepts are key to succeeding in these courses.

In biochemistry, for instance, you may have to read 200 pages of your textbook. The exam that follows will consist of questions from a number of these pages. In order to score well on your exam, you should aim to know everything on those pages.

The study technique for these courses is based on the same basic principle underlying many of the other study methods: repetition. The first time you start reading the text, you typically won't remember much. It can also be difficult to get a deep understanding of what you have read. This will likely be true for you on the second and even third rounds of repetition. This sometimes frustrates and demotivates students because they think that they will never adequately learn the content. However, the more often you read the material, the easier it will be to follow, understand, and remember the text. You will also obtain a greater understanding of the details of the content with increasing repetition. Your biggest challenge is to ensure that you do not skip any sections until you fully understand the theories behind everything you have read. By using this strategy, you will get much better acquainted with the information and remember it better.

Step by Step

1. Find out exactly what will be covered on your upcoming exam. You want to know the exact page numbers, chapters, problems to solve, tasks to do, and other things you will be tested on. Feel free to ask the teacher what they think is important, since there will always be high-yield content in every course. Moreover, go back to review all the lecture notes and make sure you include these in your preparation. Identify any areas that your teacher described as important and make sure you read these a few extra times.

2. Make a plan. Go back to Chapter 6 on time management and create a structured plan for your exam(s). You should plan to review the text five or six times depending on your ability to retain information. At the very least, you should plan to review the material a minimum of three times.

3. Start by organizing each section. For instance, DNA replication, stages of mitosis, citric acid cycle, and so on. You need to structure your studying. Typically, your textbook will provide this structure for you, so it's okay to follow it (or your lecture notes). Whatever structure you do choose, make sure you have an organized plan in terms of what content to dig into first, second, third, and so on.

4. Start reading each page for a given section and get an overview of the information. Here, you should read the book, lecture notes, and all the other material that is relevant to that specific area or section. Remember that it's normal if you don't remember or understand everything the first time through.

5. Continue to the next section and read it until you reach the end of that section or chapter.

6. Next, you will start doing questions and quizzes. At the end of a chapter, there are usually questions and problems to solve. Solve all questions that come at the end of a chapter. Highlight questions that you're not able to answer on your own and move on. Don't worry if you don't know the answers to all the questions in the beginning—after all, you've read the text only once. When you are answering the questions and solving the problems, try to understand what information and concepts the book emphasizes, since the questions at the end of the chapter are typically high-yield.

7. Continue reading the next chapter or section, and do the questions for that particular section. Continue reading all the sections until you have covered all the content you are expected to learn.

8. Once you have finished going through all the assigned chapters and pages in your textbook, your lecture notes, and other relevant materials once, read all the material again. Try to understand and actively pick up more details. Do not highlight any text just yet; your brain is still working to get the overall picture. If you start highlighting at this stage, you will highlight too much.

9. Solve all the problems and answer all the questions again. Write down all the answers in a document on your computer or in your notebook and continue to highlight questions that you are still unable to answer.

10. Start reading everything again. At this stage, you should be able to remember and understand the information better. Start by digging into important facts, high-yield knowledge, content that is harder to understand, or material that you notice is more difficult for you to remember.

11. Solve all the questions one more time. This time around, try to make sure you can answer the questions you couldn't previously. Although you may not be able to answer everything, progress is key, and you should be able to answer more and more each time.

12. Read all the content a fourth time. Highlight material that you still haven't remembered or grasped.

13. After your fourth round of repetition, review the sections you highlighted and memorize them step by step. Use the memorization techniques explained in this book.

14. Start answering all the questions once more. This will be the fourth time you are doing the questions. Most of the questions should be familiar to you, and you should be able to answer about 80% of them correctly. Pay extra attention to the questions you highlighted earlier.

15. Read the text again. At this stage, you'll notice that your comprehension and memory of the content are more solid. During this round, your memory of the answers to the questions will be strengthened too, since you will start to connect the questions to the content

in the textbook and lecture notes. Because you already know the answers quite well, your brain will now also pick up on more details in the text.

16. Solve the questions a fifth time.

17. At this stage, you have repeated your review of the text at least five times and also answered all the questions five times. You'll notice that you have good knowledge of the content. To optimize your command of the material, we will add retrieval practice, as I explained in Chapter 11 on memorization and learning techniques. Start by going back to the first section and reading the subtitle only. Now, describe the text to yourself, in your own words, without reading the content. After you are done, read the text and notice which parts you were correct about and which parts you missed or were incorrect about. Then start reviewing the next section and so on until you are done with all the content[1-3].

18. Read all the content a sixth time. This time around, make sure you have understood and memorized each section before moving on. Otherwise, *stop and learn it.*

19. Describe the content to yourself the same way you did in step 17. At this stage, if you have followed all the steps accurately, you should know at least 90% of the content.

20. Answer all questions again. At this point, make sure you understand them and know them by heart.

21. This step is not necessary, but if you have time, find another book or text with similar content and questions, then start reading the text and answering the questions.

22. Right before your exam, skim through all the content once more for a final round of repetition. Try to capture the remaining details, making sure that you know more than 90% of all the content and that you have a full understanding of it.

Summary

This chapter has presented a general guideline that works for most students studying biochemistry, cell biology, genetics, and biology courses. If you have many pages of material to read for the exam, make sure to start early so that you can repeat your review of the content as many times as needed to learn all the information. You might be a student who can comprehend the information in these courses much more quickly than others. Or you could be a student who feels that six rounds of repetition is not enough for you to confidently learn and remember the material. In that case, you will need to continue reading the content until the information is firmly implanted in your memory.

We all have different abilities, so you will need to use your common sense and be honest with yourself with respect to when you have actually learned over 90% of the content. Furthermore, if you feel that you know more than 90% of the content after the third or fourth round of repetition, then do not do additional rounds. I do not want you to waste your time; however, it is important that you understand that it frequently requires many rounds of repetition to remember and understand most of the content.

If there is content that you do not understand even after several readings, it's best to ask another student or your teacher to explain it to you. The study technique for biochemistry, cell biology, genetics, and biology courses is largely based on understanding the content well, so make sure that you make understanding your top priority. Finally, the more you read strategically and repeat, the faster and more easily your brain will recall the information, and the better you will know and understand most of the content.

References

1. Sleister H. Evidence-based strategies to improve memory and learning. *J Microbiol Biol Educ.* 2014;15(2):336–337. https://doi.org/10.1128/jmbe.v15i2.790.

2. Augustin M. How to learn effectively in medical school: test yourself, learn actively, and repeat in intervals. *Yale J Biol Med.* 2014;87(2):207–212.
3. Wolyniak MJ, Bemis LT, Prunuske AJ. Improving medical students' knowledge of genetic disease: a review of current and emerging pedagogical practices. *Adv Med Educ Pract.* 2015;6:597–607. https://doi.org/10.2147/AMEP.S73644.

CHAPTER 17

Immunology, Embryology, Pathology, Microbiology, and Physiology Courses

Introduction

Immunology, embryology, pathology, microbiology, and physiology courses have several things in common. They are usually long courses with a lot of information to read and understand. Without a doubt, the details are important, but even more important are the theories behind everything. Once you are a physician, you may not remember every single detail of the anatomy of the kidney, but you will have a good understanding of what a kidney does and why it is considered a vital organ.

The study strategy presented to you here is good for any topics where you need to read a lot of information and understand the underlying theories. One might argue that all courses in medicine require such an approach. While you do need to understand everything you study in medical school, these specific courses require even more comprehension. You need to be able to connect different bits of information, see the flow in the various processes, and understand both the big picture and the small one to understand things at their core.

Most of the questions you will see on the exam will based on the content you will have read. You will be tested on the different functions of the cells of the immune system, the function of the cardiac chambers, how a nerve impulse works, and so on. You will have to read, reread, learn, and comprehend a mountain of information to develop a good grasp of it. It's all about reading and rereading the information until it sticks.

Remember that the first time you read the chapters in the textbook, it is unlikely that you will remember much. Nor will you come away with a deep understanding either. Even during the second round of repetition, it can be tricky to remember and comprehend the content fully. But the more you read the text, the easier it will be to follow the content, catch the details, and ultimately understand and master the information. Hence, study technique 3 is similar to study technique 2 with a few differences, as you will make note of in the following step-by-step instructions. I will explain this study technique using physiology as the example.

Step by Step

1. Find out exactly what will be covered on your upcoming exam. You will need to know the exact page numbers, chapters, problems, tasks, and anything else you are expected to know and understand. Feel free to ask the teacher what they think is important as well, since there will always be high-yield content in every course. Go back to all your lecture notes and make sure you include these in your preparation. Try to identify any areas that your teacher described as important, and make sure you read these a few extra times.

2. Make a plan. Go back to Chapter 6 on time management and create a structured plan for your exam(s). You should plan to review all the content five or six times depending on your ability to retain information. At the very least, you should plan to review it a minimum of three times.

3. Start by organizing each section. For instance, you could begin with cardiac physiology, then gastrointestinal physiology, then neurophysiology, then live physiology, and so on. You need structure in your studies. Typically, your textbook will provide this structure for you, so it's okay to follow it (or your lecture notes). Whatever structure you choose, make sure you have an organized plan in terms of what to dig into first, second, third, and so on.

4. Start reading each page for a given section and get an overview of the information. Here, you should read the book, lecture notes, and all the other material that is relevant for that section. Remember that it's normal if you don't remember or understand everything the first time through.

5. Continue to the next section and read it until you reach the end of that section or chapter.

6. Read the text a second time. Try to understand and actively pick up more details. Do not highlight anything yet: your brain is still working to get the overall picture. If you start highlighting at this stage, you will highlight too much.

7. Now, reread everything a third time. At this point, you should be able to remember and understand things better. Start digging into important facts, high-yield knowledge, content that is harder to understand, and material that you notice is more difficult to remember. During this round of repetition, you will also begin to emphasize the information and concepts that are extra important and the more detailed material that needs to be memorized.

8. Since these courses require that you have a strong command of the content, I want you to read the text three times before you start answering any questions. Otherwise, it may be a waste of your time because you don't yet have a strong enough understanding. Now, start answering questions related to your exam. Answer all the questions and solve all the problems related to the chapter or topic. Highlight questions you are not able to answer on your own and move on. Don't worry if you can't answer all the questions in the beginning—after all, you have read the text only once. When you are solving the problems and answering the questions, try to understand what information and concept the textbook emphasizes, since the questions at the end of the chapter are typically high-yield.

9. Read all the content a fourth time. Highlight information that you still haven't remembered or grasped.

10. Once you have finished your fourth round of repetition, review the sections you highlighted and memorize them step by step. Use the memorization techniques explained in this book.

11. Start answering all the questions once more. Pay extra attention to the questions you highlighted earlier.

12. Read the text for a fifth time. At this stage, you'll notice that your comprehension and memory of the content are more solid. During this round, your memory of the answers to the questions will be strengthened too, since you will start to connect the questions to the

content in the textbook or lecture notes. Because you already know the answers quite well, your brain will now also pick up on more details in the text.

13. Solve all the questions a third time.

14. Now it's time for retrieval practice[1-3]. Start by going back to the first section and reading only the subtitle. Next, describe the text to yourself, in your own words, without reading the content. After you are done, read the text and notice which parts you were correct about and which parts you missed or were incorrect about. Then start with the next section and so on until you are done with all the content.

15. Start answering all the questions once more. This will be the fourth time you are going through the questions. Most of the questions should be familiar to you, and you should be able to answer about 80% correctly.

16. Read the entire text a sixth time. This time around, make sure you have understood and memorized each section before moving on. Otherwise, *stop and learn it*.

17. Describe the content to yourself the same way you did in step 14. At this stage, if you have followed all the steps accurately, you should know about 90% or more of the content.

18. Solve all the questions a fifth time. Make sure you understand and know them by heart.

19. This step is not necessary, but if you have time, find another book or text with similar content and questions, then start reading the text and answering the questions.

20. Right before your exam, skim through all the pages once more for a final round of repetition. Try to capture the last details, making sure you know more than 90% of all the content and have a full understanding of it.

Summary

This chapter has presented a general guideline for students wishing to comprehend immunology, embryology, pathology, microbiology, and physiology courses. Your comprehension is important not just for your successful exam performance, but also for your future career as a physician. You may get the impression that reading the text this many times is redundant. Perhaps it is for you, and perhaps it is not. You should invest your time in thoroughly understanding all the content, however many rounds of repetition it takes. However, if you feel that you know and understand 90% of the content and can answer all questions after only three rounds of repetition, then that is your golden number. We are all different, and it is up to you to decide when you feel confident in your knowledge of a subject.

References

1. Sleister H. Evidence-based strategies to improve memory and learning. *J Microbiol Biol Educ.* 2014;15(2):336–337. https://doi.org/10.1128/jmbe.v15i2.790.
2. Augustin M. How to learn effectively in medical school: test yourself, learn actively, and repeat in intervals. *Yale J Biol Med.* 2014;87(2):207–212.
3. Wolyniak MJ, Bemis LT, Prunuske AJ. Improving medical students' knowledge of genetic disease: a review of current and emerging pedagogical practices. *Adv Med Educ Pract.* 2015;6:597–607. https://doi.org/10.2147/AMEP.S73644.

Ethics and Behavioral Science Courses

Introduction

Ethics and behavioral science courses will form a smaller part of your medical education but they are still just as important to learn and comprehend. These subjects are critical in medicine and in your future career as a physician. You will encounter numerous ethical issues no matter what specialty you pursue, and knowing how to deal with these issues is key. In your training, you will learn how people make decisions and behave, which can then help you to draw conclusions and make predictions. These courses are interesting, and in my experience and that of many other students, most of the exam questions are not very difficult as long as you know the concepts. The most important thing is to understand the topics and be able to apply them to real- life scenarios. This chapter provides you with a step-by-step approach to learning the material in your ethics and behavioral science courses.

Step by Step

1. As with all study techniques, the first step is always to find out exactly what material will be covered on your upcoming exam. Identify the exact page numbers, chapters, problems, tasks, and other things you are expected to know. Feel free to ask the teacher what they think is important, since there will always be high-yield content in every course. Moreover, go back to all the lecture notes and make sure you include these as part of your preparation. Try to find all areas that your teacher described as important, and make sure you read these a few extra times.
2. Make a plan. Go back to Chapter 6 on time management and create a structured plan for your exam(s). You should plan to repeat your review of all the text at least three times.
3. Organize each section that you need to review for your exam. You can follow your textbook or your lecture notes. Identify what you need to review first, second, third, and so on.
4. Start reading each page for that particular section and get an overview of the information. You should read the book, lecture notes, and any other material that is relevant for that specific section.
5. Review each section until you have finished reviewing all the sections you need to cover for the exam.

6. At the end of each chapter and section, there are often questions and problems to solve. Or your teacher may have given you questions and problems to solve. Solve all the questions that are related to the exam once. Highlight questions that you are unable to answer on your own and move on. Don't worry if you don't know all the answers in the beginning because you have read the text just one time. When you are solving the questions and problems, try to get an understanding of what material the book has emphasized, since the questions that follow are typically high-yield.

7. Read the text again. Try to understand and pick up more details.

8. Solve all the questions and problems again. Write the answers down in your computer or notebook and continue to highlight questions you are still unable to answer.

9. Now it's time to analyze the concepts. Try to compare (identify similarities and differences), examine, experiment with, organize, and question the material you have learned. By looking at the concepts in different ways, you are using different areas of your brain to connect the dots and see beyond the knowledge presented. This step will allow you to remember the text much better as well. You can do this alone or with another student.

10. Start re-reading the material. At this point, you should be remembering things better and gaining a deeper understanding. Also dig into important facts, high-yield knowledge, concepts that are harder to understand, and material that you notice is more difficult to remember.

11. Solve all the problems and answer all the questions again. This time around, try to make sure you are able to answer the questions you previously couldn't. Although you may not be able to answer every single question, progress is key: you should be able to answer even more at this stage.

12. Start applying the concepts in new situations: execute, implement, demonstrate, solve, use, and interpret the knowledge in real-life scenarios. For example, think about a challenging patient situation you observed or a family member that was sick. Whatever you do, be sure to apply the knowledge you have learned to real situations. Ask yourself, What would you do if this particular situation came up? You can do this exercise with another student or by yourself.

13. Now it's time for retrieval practice[1-3]. Imagine yourself being the professor or teacher of the class. Start by going back to the first section and reading only the subtitle. Now, explain the ideas or concepts to yourself or to a friend: describe, identify, recognize, translate, and discuss the different sections to yourself, in your own words, without reading the content. After you are done describing the text to yourself, read the text to identify which parts you explained correctly and whether you missed or were incorrect about any material. Then, go to the next section and repeat the process until you have gone through all the content.

14. If you need to, read the entire text one more time. Make sure you have understood and memorized each section before you move on. Otherwise, *stop and learn it.*

15. At this point, if you are still struggling with some of the problems or questions, review them again and make sure to understand them and know them by heart before moving on.

16. Right before your exam, skim through all the pages one last time for a final round of repetition. Try to capture any final important details. Make sure you know and thoroughly understand more than 90% of all the content.

References

1. Sleister H. Evidence-based strategies to improve memory and learning. *J Microbiol Biol Educ.* 2014;15(2):336–337. https://doi.org/10.1128/jmbe.v15i2.790.

2. Augustin M. How to learn effectively in medical school: test yourself, learn actively, and repeat in intervals. *Yale J Biol Med.* 2014;87(2):207–212.
3. Wolyniak MJ, Bemis LT, Prunuske AJ. Improving medical students' knowledge of genetic disease: a review of current and emerging pedagogical practices. *Adv Med Educ Pract.* 2015;6:597–607. https://doi.org/10.2147/AMEP.S73644.

Clinical Rotations

Introduction

In medical school, you will participate in many different clinical rotations and clinical exams. Most of your third year will consist of rotations in surgery, family medicine, pediatrics, obstetrics and gynecology, psychiatry, and internal medicine. During your fourth year, you may also have rotations in anesthesiology, radiology, neurology, and emergency medicine. Your clinical rotations will be slightly different depending on your medical school's curriculum, rotations they offer, and your choice of electives/clerkships and sub-internships. These rotations will be graded, and you will be expected to perform well by demonstrating both your theoretical knowledge and your social skills.

Social and emotional skills are critical here. The way you come across, how you interact with others, whether you are pleasant (or not), whether you are helpful, whether you come across as interested, ambitious, and well balanced—these all play a role in your clinical evaluations. I know of many smart students who did not do well on the residency match or were not invited to many interviews strictly because of their lack of social and emotional skills. The most important thing is to know as much as possible about the specialty that you are rotating in, know the patients that you are taking care of, be kind and pleasant, communicate well with others, and help out as much as you can. You need to show your evaluators that you are a hard worker and genuinely interested in this field. Below are specific tips on how to perform well.

Step by Step

1. **Learn the field as well as you can.** Let's say you are starting your clinical rotation in general surgery. You know that general surgery has different fields, including colorectal surgery, transplant surgery, endocrine surgery, and more. The way you learn the theoretical aspects of those different sections is by reading the books on the most common disorders that you will be encountering during your rotation. You learn this theoretical knowledge through the study techniques I previously shared with you. Just remember that before any clinical rotation, your knowledge should be on point. You must demonstrate that you have studied the different diseases and management of certain conditions extremely well so that when you are asked questions, you know most of the answers. Make reading and comprehending the theoretical knowledge for each specialty your top priority. You should make an ongoing effort to read and learn throughout each rotation.

2. **Arrive at your clinical rotations early in the morning.** You have to know about all the patients you are taking care of. And the only way to do that is to arrive early and read up on the patients. Sometimes you might have 20 to 30 patients, if not more, in your care. Although you are not expected to manage all of them, you will likely get assigned to take care of a few. However, in the first few days, you should make a conscious effort to get to know as much as you can about every single patient. This will make a huge difference when you are evaluated. Things to know about each patient (and take notes so you don't forget) are the following:

   - Why the patient is in the hospital? What happened?
   - Past medical history
   - Past surgical history
   - Social history
   - Family history
   - Medications
   - Overnight events: What happened from the time the team left the hospital until you came in?
   - Vital signs
   - Relevant laboratory results
   - Any workup or tests that were performed
   - Talk to and examine your patient: What are their subjective complaints? How was the physical exam?
   - Assessment of this patient
   - Your plan

3. **Be prepared to present patients.** As a medical student, you are expected to present patients to your residents and sometimes even to your attendings. You want to present the overnight events, subjective complaints of the patient, vital signs, laboratory results, test results, physical exam, your assessment, and then your plan. Everyone likes their presentations done differently, and presentation style could differ from specialty to specialty. It's best to *ask* your team, your chief resident, or perhaps even your attending what structure of presentation they prefer and then follow that structure. But whatever you do, make sure your presentation is on point and that you do not look at the paper. You should know all the labs, vital signs, and events in your head and present in a calm and confident manner. The presentation cannot be too long either. It's a fine balance. You also need to ensure that you always have an accurate plan for your patients. If you aren't sure, ask or find out. This is your time to start developing your analytical skills and learning how to devise a management plan for your patients; the better you are at this, the smarter you will come across and the better your evaluations will be.

4. **Bring supplies with you to rounds.** Oftentimes you will need to change dressings, remove sutures, or listen to the heart and lungs. Make sure that you have all the supplies you need and anything that the team for that rotation needs. The more you can show that you are an asset to the team, the better. Always bring your stethoscope, flashlight, reflex hammer, and other essential items that the specialty you are rotating with always brings with them.

5. **Be reliable and competent.** There is no better way to prove yourself than to demonstrate that you know things that others do not. Knowledge is power. If a question comes up on rounds such as "Does the patient have a cardiologist?" or "What is their baseline creatinine level?", and you know the answer, then you will certainly be valued more highly. Know *everything* there is to know about each patient: previous hospital stays, past medical history, past surgical history, current medications, and so on. To your evaluators, it is a sign that you are well prepared and competent. Of course, this level of competence takes time to develop, but my general tip is that you need to get obsessed with data and information. I used to

come 1 to 2 hours before rounds began just to learn as much as I could about every single patient. This effort paid off tremendously.

6. **Be hard-working and pleasant.** No one wants to work with a lazy or unpleasant person. Imagine the high regard you would have for a friendly and diligent medical student; be that person. Being pleasant takes you far. Always say hello and goodbye, ask whether you can help out with anything, and be enthusiastic about the field. If someone shouts at you or gets mad, do not get defensive. Instead, be calm, swallow it, and say, "Thanks for the feedback, I will do better!" As for working hard: Arrive early, leave late, and show your evaluators that you are not trying to escape from work. Assist your team members with anything they need help with, and come back to see patients regularly for status updates that the team may need but does not have time for because they are busy. This way, you will also build relationships with patients, who may leave great reviews of you with your team.

Social Skills and Emotional Intelligence

Social skills and emotional intelligence are extremely important skills to master not just to do well in school but in life[1-3]. In short, these are skills that enable people to develop and maintain healthy communication, behavior, and relationships. When you use these skills, you increase your productivity, performance, and long-term success in school and life.

Here are some of the important skills that you should develop and practice in your clinical rotations:

- **Self-awareness.** This is key. Self-awareness is the conscious knowledge of one's character, feelings, weaknesses, motives, and desires. It is our ability to track our thoughts, emotions, beliefs, and inner world. The way you become self-aware is to examine yourself. Be aware of how you are doing and how you feel at all times. Think about how you come across when you talk; when you're not talking, think about the things you say, how you say them, how you feel, and so on. Analyze the feedback you receive from others in terms of your way of being, and adjust your inner attitude and behavior based on that information. Be as honest and nonjudgmental toward yourself as possible. Self-compassion is also key. We all have good and bad traits, but many people are largely unaware of what these are. The more self-aware you become, the more easily you can identify those traits. You will be able to strengthen the good ones and minimize or eliminate the bad ones. How you feel inside also dictates the way you behave and respond to others. If you are in a negative frame of mind or not feeling well and you can identify that you feel this way, you can prevent poor communication and inappropriate responses to others just through your awareness.

- **Empathy.** Everyone has their own struggles, often without our knowing about them. Many people are tired, frustrated, and stressed out. Empathy is all about feeling with another person's experience even though you may not always know what that experience is like. Step out of your own world and try to feel for what others are going through. By taking on another person's perspective and experience, you will in turn behave differently towards them. Everyone has a deep need to feel seen, heard, and understood. Showing that you have empathy builds intimacy, trust, and thus deeper relationships.

- **Emotional regulation.** There will be days when you, too, will feel tired, stressed, angry, frustrated, sad, and so on. In those situations, it is easy to react or behave in a way that comes across as impolite, impatient, or unkind. However, practicing emotional regulation will make you more mature and give you better control in challenging situations. Being mindful of your feelings allows you to start adding a pause between your feelings and your knee-jerk reactions. With increased self-control, you will gain the ability to remain calm under pressure and prevent yourself from behaving inappropriately and against your values.

- **Communication.** This is a huge topic that we cannot give justice to in the space we have here. Just remember that there are specific strategies to communicate well. And that *what* you say and *how* you say it will affect how others see you. Communication is something you can spend your entire life improving.
- **Understanding others.** You can begin to understand others by learning how to recognize cues in others' behaviors: their tone of voice, their body language, and their facial expressions are the key things to pay attention to. Try to get a sense of how the other person is feeling and try to improve, or at least not worsen, their emotional state in all settings. This will make them trust and like you much more.
- **Listening.** Listen deeply. Be all ears. While most people like to talk, they generally do not want to listen. Thus, if you listen more than you talk, you are giving others the thing that they want: the chance to talk. Poor listeners are not looked upon well. Furthermore, the more you listen, the more you learn.

Why did I write this section? Because in medicine, you will work with people—many, many people. And your grades and evaluations will largely depend on how well you are liked by others. Many residency programs pick candidates mainly according to how well they get along with others. Most students in medicine are smart and hard-working; that's a fact. However, not many can get along with different types of personalities. If your evaluator doesn't like you, then chances are that you will perform poorly and vice versa. Therefore, learning better social skills is essential and something you should master. You can read a lot more about how to master social skills and emotional intelligence in the many books that have been published on the subject.

References

1. Goleman D. *Emotional Intelligence: Why It Can Matter More Than IQ*. Bantam Books; 1995.
2. Czabanowska K, Malho A, Schröder-Bäck P, Popa D, Burazeri G. Do we develop public health leaders? Association between public health competencies and emotional intelligence: a cross-sectional study. *BMC Med Educ*. 2014;14:83. https://doi.org/10.1186/1472-6920-14-83.
3. Naeem N, van der Vleuten C, Muijtjens AM, et al. Correlates of emotional intelligence: results from a multi-institutional study among undergraduate medical students. *Med Teach*. 2014;36(Suppl. 1):S30–S35. https://doi.org/10.3109/0142159X.2014.886008.

Practical Courses

Introduction

Medicine is a clinical profession. Most physicians will see and take care of patients or perform tasks that have clinical relevance. Some courses in medical school also require practical knowledge that you will acquire on your clinical rotations, such as learning how to suture. To be good at something practical, you have to do it over and over again as many times as you can. When a dentist has performed over 100 root canal fillings, then he knows he can perform that procedure very well. When a surgeon has operated on over 200 gallbladders, then she knows she can perform those surgeries very well. However, before performing a root canal or operating on a gallbladder, a dentist or a surgeon must first learn the theories behind these procedures. In the same way, you must first learn the theoretical background of any practical procedure you intend to perform. Once you know the theories, you can start to practice the procedure to understand what to do, when and how to do it, and why.

In practical courses, there is a systematic way to do things. Doing something well is not a matter of performing random actions. That's why we do residency training in surgery, for instance—so that we can learn techniques that others have already done many times before and have developed in a systematic fashion. Thus, the first step after learning the theories is to learn the systematic way of doing each procedure: each step, technique, and method involved. Once you have gained this knowledge, you can begin practicing it over and over again to develop those skills, fine tune them, and optimize them.

You don't need to think about speed in the beginning. First, you need to learn how to do something the right way. Then you need to learn how to do it well. Finally, you need to learn how to do it well, as fast as possible. But speed should never jeopardize quality.

Step by Step

1. Learn the theory behind the practical course you are taking. If you are learning how to suture, study books about suturing, different suture materials, suture techniques, and so on. Watch videos and try to get a sense of what suturing is all about, as well as what to do and how and when to do it. Try to understand why this is done the way it is, and think about why it is done in that specific order.
2. Next, you will likely be taught how to do what you are going to learn to do. Pay attention to the teacher's demonstration. Listen carefully, take notes, and write down a description

of each step. Remember: Write down each step in your own words. Even if you think you will remember it later, you should always write it down so that you can return to your notes and confirm what you need to do. Furthermore, never miss a demonstration and think you can learn it yourself. You may be able to learn how to do something by reading books and watching videos, but oftentimes there are multiple ways of doing one thing; the way your teacher is showing you is the way they want you to learn to do it. You will never get a coherent picture of a procedure and know exactly how to do it in practice until you have observed it in reality.

3. Now it is time to practice. Start by practicing what you are going to do step by step. Do not rush it. Again, don't think about speed. Just try to learn the correct, systematic way of doing it. Try to memorize each step, and think about the theories behind each step in your mind as you are doing them. Practice as many times as you can and go slowly. In the beginning, it is all about doing the procedure the right way. If you miss any steps or get stuck, go back to your notes, review some videos, or ask someone to help you get it right.

4. Return to your notes and read the theories once more. This step will further optimize your practical abilities. Once you know how to do something and have practiced it a few times, reading about the "how," "when," and "why" will solidify your practical knowledge.

5. Review your demonstration notes and read all the steps again. Make sure that you are doing all the steps required and build a mental image of how you are going to perform this procedure, step by step. Visualization will make it easier to remember all the steps as you are doing them.

6. Practice more. Practice, practice, practice. Make sure you practice until every step is clear and you have a flow in what you want to do. Sometimes, you have to practice something 10 times and sometimes 100 times each day before you become good at it. And since you are expecting to achieve the best grade and evaluation possible, you should practice doing things well. It all comes down to practice. The more you do it, the better you will be.

7. Write down any questions you have regarding your practical course, experience, or test and bring them to your teacher. Questions always come up when you are trying to learn something new. The best approach is to write them down after you have practiced the procedure for a while and then ask your teacher for clarification.

8. Practice in your head. Every night, before you go to bed or when you have some down time, visualize all the steps you are going to perform. Practicing the steps in your head will help to strengthen your memory of how to perform the procedures.

9. Practice more. This time around, try to anticipate the next step before you get to it. You should practice until you feel that your performance comes naturally, without any hesitation.

10. Finally, *teach* others what you have learned to do. Remember the traditional method of medical learning: "See one, do one, teach one"; this method is still applicable[1]. Teach it to a classmate, a parent, or someone else who is willing to listen and can ask simple questions. Show them exactly how each step is done and explain why. When you have done it a few times, you will have developed your ability to confidently convey what you have learned to someone else, and then you can do the procedure confidently when the real test arrives.

Final Tips

During tests of your practical skills, your teacher wants to see that you are independent and can perform the task safely and easily with good flow. They don't want to see any hesitation or disruption. The great thing about practical learning is that it all comes to you with practice. The more you practice, the better you will do it. Trust me on this. Just as you know how to brush your teeth or type on a computer without thinking about it, you should know how to perform any practical procedure, step by step, just by doing it over and over again.

Reference

1. Kotsis SV, Chung KC. Application of the "see one, do one, teach one" concept in surgical training. *Plast Reconstr Surg.* 2013;131(5):1194–1201. https://doi.org/10.1097/PRS.0b013e318287a0b3.

Reports and Assignments

Introduction

In medical school, you will often be required to submit assignments or reports. These need to be professionally and accurately written. A strategic approach to writing will elevate your reports and assignments, demonstrating your analytical abilities and ultimately giving you a high grade.

The most important thing to remember about these assignments and reports is that they be accurate, follow the teacher's rule and instructions, and show your capacity to analyze and draw your own conclusions based on what you have learned. A report, essay, or any other type of submission should not just be a summary of a text that you have read from an article or a book because anyone can do that. Therefore, make sure you follow most if not all of these steps when you draft these reports.

Step by Step

1. **Find out what is expected.** The first step is to find out exactly what you need to do. Don't just aim for a general idea of what you need to submit. Determine exactly what you need to write about, and listen closely to how the teacher wants you to write the report or assignment. Most often your teacher wants you to do something specific. If you receive a document containing written instructions, then read them carefully. Follow the teacher's verbal or written instructions religiously and make sure you understand the assignment to the core. If you're not sure, ask!

2. **Gather information.** Now that you understand what you need to do, start gathering information about the subject. Look into books, course literature, online material, videos, and so on. For example, if you want to write about antibiotics, then first you need to gather all the information you can. Do not start to write anything yet.

3. **Organize the information.** Let's say you are going to write a report about antibiotics. Obviously, you are not going to write everything about antibiotics, as you most likely have specific directions about what to write about within a given topic and also have a limited word count. Therefore, after you have found your resources, you should organize your content, structure it, include the necessary information, and exclude irrelevant information. Carefully review your resources and decide what is important and what you want to include in your report. You can do this by highlighting pages, text, sections, adding and removing references, and saving websites on your computer.

4. **Make a plan.** As you've likely heard before, failing to plan is planning to fail. Similar to making a study plan for an exam, you must now make a plan for what you are going to write. What is your direction and focus? What comes first? What comes second? What part of the information you collected should be included, and how should you divide your work into different sections? How should the information be included in a relevant way? How are you going to structure and organize the work? Will you include any images? What should be where? Always ask yourself *why* you are going to include something; if you do not have a good answer, do not include it. Your content must always have a purpose and be accurate. In medical school, it also needs to be supported by scientific evidence. You cannot merely add your own opinion or whatever information you find online. Thus, make sure that you cite scientific references for any statements you make.

5. **Start writing.** Now, you can finally start to write your report or assignment. Write your text based on your plan and according to your teacher's instructions. Write professionally and in an interesting way. Always write in your own words, and do not copy and paste from other resources. Finish all the sections you need to write in an organized manner. Remember that a text should always be structured and easy for a reader to follow. Add titles and subtitles where needed. Illustrate important or complicated information with images and diagrams.

6. **Analyze and discuss.** Discuss your topic, reflect on it, and draw conclusions. This is where the grade usually differs between students. Connect your main topic to other topics, and explore whether you can find similarities and differences that are logical and interesting. Ask whether there are differences and similarities with other fields and consider what they would look like. Is there anything positive or negative about your topic? Why? How does this affect us as people and patients? The community? The future? The medical field? What opinions do you have about what you have written? Do you have ideas on what can be done better in the future? Come up with new ideas! In what way does your opinion resemble those of others? How does your opinion differ? These are just a few questions that will take you far each time you write something. The teacher wants to know whether you have an analytical mind and can discuss your topic "outside the box."

7. **Review your work.** Read through your work at least three times. Spelling and grammatical errors will lower your grade, so make sure that you check for any errors (spelling, grammar, incorrect references, etc.). There are always things you might have missed, spelling and grammatical errors you can fix, or sentences that could be more clearly worded. Be critical of your own text. Is it written well? Did you include all the sections you needed to? Check your instruction sheet one more time to make sure of this. Should something be added or removed? Are there words or sentences in the text where you are unsure of the spelling or grammar? Have you written an interesting discussion and conclusion?

8. **Have someone else read your paper.** It could be a sibling, your parents, or a friend. Choose someone who is reasonably knowledgeable about medicine and/or the topic so that they can correct or improve your paper. Think of someone who could further enhance your paper and hopefully make it better—perhaps a senior medical student. However, avoid asking your classmates unless you write the report together. Ask whoever is reviewing your paper to be critical and provide feedback that will improve your paper.

9. **Revise your paper.** After you have received feedback from someone you know, revise your report or assignment according to their comments. Make sure that you think critically about the other person's remarks. Sometimes people say things that don't make sense, so it's up to you to discern what does and does not seem appropriate.

10. **Reread your paper.** Read your work one last time to make sure you're satisfied with what you have written.

Final Tips

To write just what the teacher is asking for will probably result in a passing grade. To get top scores and the best grades, you have to write a thoughtful discussion and reach valid and valuable conclusions. Only then will have you demonstrated that you can analyze a topic with a critical mind. The truth is that anyone can research information on a topic and write about it, but only a few can investigate and explore a topic well.

What your discussion and conclusion consist of will depend on what you are going to write about and what the purpose of your work is. However, there are certain strategies to consider when writing your paper. Many good conclusions come from relevant comparisons with other fields and topics, from differences and similarities with other phenomena. When you start to research your paper, you will not yet be able to make comparisons. But as you learn more about the topic, you can start thinking more creatively and think about how your topic relates to other subjects. Be innovative and imaginative. Become a visionary and don't get caught up in what is—instead, consider what could be and why!

Presentations

Introduction

Presentations are a given in medical school. The two major challenges faced by most students are (1) getting over the fear of speaking in front of an audience and (2) delivering an interesting presentation. Many students do not like to speak in front of others. This fear of public speaking has a cure: it's called practice. As with any other fears or phobias, the most important thing is to expose yourself to the thing you are afraid of. Doing so will slowly desensitize you.

If you have a phobia of spiders, for instance, the worst thing you can do is to avoid them altogether. That will never lessen your fear. However, if you start looking at spiders, touching spiders, reading about spiders, and ultimately holding spiders, your brain will realize that most spiders are not dangerous and that the fear you feel is just a cortical creation.

Similarly, you become more comfortable with speaking in public the more you get to know your classmates. We all know that we are more comfortable talking in front of people we know. The longer you are in your class and the better you get to know your classmates, the less shy you will be when the time comes to give a presentation.

As for a good presentation, you can increase your chances of giving one by delivering the material in a creative and enthusiastic manner.

Step by Step

1. **Overcome your fear of public speaking.** A good speaker is confident, charismatic, and articulate and speaks with conviction, in a way that makes people want to listen. A good speaker affects people. To become that kind of speaker, you have to overcome your fear of public speaking. Most people are nervous at first, but that fades with practice. Yes, you heard it right—practice is the key. The more you speak in front of people, the better you will get and the faster your fear will disappear. Look up articles and videos on how to speak in public and start practicing today. Also, absolutely everyone feels nervous at the beginning of a presentation; that nervousness subsides shortly after the presentation has started. Remembering that basic fact will help you to mentally prepare. Go ahead and speak in front of others even if it feels uncomfortable or unnatural. Every time you do it, it will get easier and you will feel more comfortable. With enough presentations under your belt, you might discover that you love doing it!

2. **Be well prepared.** The more you know about your topic, the better you will be able to speak on it and the more confident you will feel and appear. Read up on the topic you are going to present about until you know it well. A good speaker knows their topic inside and out. As a result, you will appear confident and knowledgeable to your listeners. Note any points you think are important and that you want to bring up in your talk.

3. **Organize your presentation.** Structure all the information you want to include in your presentation. Make sure you know what you are going to include first, second, third, and so on. A presentation needs to be organized. Most presentations are done in Microsoft PowerPoint. If this is the software you are using, then make sure your slides are clean, well designed, and easy to follow. Do not include too much text per slide. Only a few bullet points should be on each slide; the rest should be content that you talk about. Always include the following points:
    - Title of the topic you are going to present, your name, title, school, etc.
    - Table of contents
    - Introduction
    - All the slides you are presenting
    - Conclusion
    - Questions
    - Acknowledgements
    - Thank you

4. **Create a visually appealing presentation.** Make your presentation visually appealing. Everyone likes to look at nice things, so the neater and nicer your presentation is, the more attention you will get. Relevant pictures, charts, tables, lists, or objects should dominate your presentation instead of plain text.

5. **Practice your presentation.** Once you have finished creating your presentation, you must practice. The more you practice, the better your presentation will be. Do not just practice twice. Practice 10 times if that is what it takes for you to feel as though you are an expert on your topic. Practice in front of the mirror or record yourself speaking. Review the recording and analyze yourself. What can you do better? Make those adjustments and practice again as many times as you need until you know everything without having to look at your paper.

6. **Practice in front of someone else.** Practice your presentation in front of someone else, maybe a sibling, parent, or friend. Ask them to give you feedback and mention everything that you can improve upon.

7. **Get ready.** Now you are ready to take center stage. Have a piece of paper that you can look at to organize your thoughts. Get there early. Dress well. Once it is your turn, get up there and look confident. Be serious and focused but smile a little so you aren't too stiff. Wait until the room gets quiet, then introduce yourself and tell everyone what you are going to talk about. The following is an example of how I introduce myself and my topic:
    - "Hello everyone. My name is Raman Mehrzad and I will now talk about common colds. I will first share a bit of information about what common colds are as well as their prevalence, incidence, etiology, symptoms, and treatment. Then I will tell you how you can prevent colds and also things you can do to boost your immune system when fever has already set in. Finally, I will show a short film clip illustrating what it looks like inside the body when microorganisms attack you, and how the immune system protects us. I will end my talk by answering any questions you may have, but you are welcome to ask questions during the presentation as well."

8. **Improve your communication skills.** As you present, keep in mind the following points about your style of communication:
    - **Gaze.** Throughout the presentation, look people right in the eyes, and shift your gaze around the room; don't just look at one person for the entire talk. Also, don't look down

at your paper or your slides, and don't look down at the floor. Try to look confident by changing who you look at every time you start a new sentence.

- **Speech.** Vary how you speak. The brain is sensitive to changes in frequency, so if your voice is constantly changing, then your audience's attention will be greater. If you maintain the same volume and pace for your entire presentation, you quickly become monotonous and risk losing people's attention. Emphasize certain words or sentences more forcefully. Never sound rushed, unclear, or disorganized.
- **Body language.** Once you start talking, be sure to use your body language as much as you can. Gesture with your arms, body, and head. If you are able to, stand while you present and walk around a little while you talk rather than standing fixed in one place.
- **Engage your audience.** Make sure you have eye contact with your class and ask questions. Engage them. Encourage them to share comments with you and ask questions, either during or at the end of the presentation. Do things that capture the audience's interest and attention. Speak with enthusiasm, charm, and charisma. Try to come across as though you truly enjoy standing there and talking, and that you are passionate about what you are saying.
- **Questions.** At the end of your presentation, make sure that you ask your audience whether they have any questions. Provide positive reinforcement by saying, "That is a great question!" Answer the question to the best of your knowledge and then ask whether there are any other questions.
- **Ending.** After all the questions have been answered, thank everyone for listening, close down your presentation, and walk back to your seat with confidence.

Final Tips

If you get disorganized, nervous, or lose your train of thought during the speech, don't panic: it happens to everyone. Just accept the flub, take a quick pause, and move on. You can also admit that you have just lost your train of thought and move on. Everyone makes mistakes and it's not the end of the world. Remember that the more you practice your talk, the less likely it is that you'll find yourself in this situation. So practice, practice, practice. Practice makes perfect!

Like a trained soldier, ready to enter the battlefield with all the necessary training, knowledge, and discipline they have learned, you are now ready to take on medical school and succeed.

You have learned the mentality, the value-based thinking, the study techniques, and the environmental factors that will make you thrive throughout your medical education.

I hope you've understood the meaning of each and every factor that plays a role in your success as a student and how it will affect your future. It will take time, energy, and a lot of hard work. But I also hope that you now truly understand that all this effort will be worth it in the end.

One day, when you are whoever you want to be and working in your dream job, you will be able to smile and be proud of what you have achieved. On that day, you will thank yourself for all the effort you put into this process.

Now that you've read this book, you have all the knowledge and tools you need to excel. If you follow my principles and methods, and if you are prepared to work hard, you really don't have to worry. Because now you know how to motivate yourself, how to set up and plan your studies, how to set goals, how to handle the surrounding environment, and how to perform optimally on your exams. In addition, you have been taught how to take care of your body with physical activity, sleep, and diet. And last but not least, you have now learned the techniques to study the right way. You have the exact recipe to follow so that you can do well each time, and learn all the knowledge you need in an effective and structured way.

Remember, however, that this is just the beginning. The knowledge of how to do something is just the start. YOU have to ultimately do the work. No one else can do it for you. Nevertheless, if you follow all the principles in this book, you will very likely succeed.

I hope that you feel ignited by genuine enthusiasm so that you have the intrinsic motivation to reach your goal and enjoy the journey along the way. Make the decision to strive for success and to want to succeed as bad as you want to breathe and I promise you that there's nothing that can stop you, no matter how tough it gets.

So go out there, start today, and chase the life you have dreamt of!

Best wishes to you!

Contact information

For questions, comments, private consultations, or lectures, contact me at:

- Email: raman_m1@hotmail.com
- Website: www.ramanmehrzad.com

And don't forget to follow me on social media for more inspiration, motivation, and knowledge about personal growth and performance:

- Instagram: @RamanMehrzad
- TikTok: RamanMehrzad
- SnapChat: RamanMehrzad
- Facebook: Raman Mehrzad
- LinkedIn: Raman Mehrzad
- Twitter: Raman Mehrzad

INDEX

Note: Page numbers followed by *f* indicate figures, *t* indicate tables, and *b* indicate boxes.